ON THE BALL:
Innovative Activities For Adult Fitness and Cardiac Rehabilitation Programs

Barry A. Franklin, Ph.D.
Director, Cardiac Rehabilitation and Exercise Laboratories
William Beaumont Hospital

Associate Professor of Physiology
Wayne State University, School of Medicine

Neil B. Oldridge, Ph.D.
Professor of Health Sciences, School of Allied Health Professions
University of Wisconsin - Milwaukee

Clinical Professor, Division of Biostatistics and Clinical Epidemiology
Medical College of Wisconsin

Professor of Physical Education and Medicine
McMaster University

Karl G. Stoedefalke, Ph.D.
Professor Exercise and Sport Sciences
Director of Health Enhancement

Executive Management Programs, College of Business Administration
The Pennsylvania State University

William E. Loechel
Medical Illustrator, Birmingham, Michigan

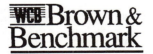

WCB Brown & Benchmark

DEDICATIONS

To my mother and father, Lottie and Norm Franklin, who taught me about values, honesty, and integrity - lessons about life that books and courses never convey.

B.A.F.

To Bruno Balke, who has all his life fostered creative and innovative physical exercise in the fight against the degenerative consequences of modern sedentary living; and to my wife, Judy Oldridge, whose patience has often been stretched.

N.B.O.

To the hundreds of exercise specialists who strive to improve the quality of life of others through physical activity.

K.G.S.

Library of Congress Publication Data:

FRANKLIN, BARRY A. 1948-

Cover Design: Gary Schmitt

Editor: Kendal Gladish

Library of Congress Catalog Card Number: 86-70734

ISBN: 0-697-14811-4

Printed in the United States of America

10 9 8 7 6 5 4 3 2

The Publisher and Authors disclaim responsibility for any adverse effects or consequences from the misapplication or injudicious use of the information contained within this text.

CONTENTS

PREFACE

"Next time you pass a children's playground, stop and listen. Hear the laughter? They're having a ball!"

Joan Lippert

Interest in the medical role of exercise as a self-improvement technique has continued to escalate. Most Americans now believe that exercise is good for them. Moreover, physicians have embraced the use of exercise in the treatment of a variety of clinical conditions and chronic health problems.

While many individuals can be encouraged to initiate an exercise program, few maintain long-term compliance. The problem? In a word, *motivation*.

Although there are many books on the scientific and theoretical basis of exercise programming and prescription, we recognized the need for, and value of, a book that would provide exercise leaders with practical ideas and clearly illustrated pleasurable activities (exercises).

The "Games-As-Aerobics" approach stresses fun, pleasure, and repeated success. Calisthenic and endurance activities are camouflaged as games, relays, or stunts, incorporating ball passing and other movement skills for variety. Game rules are often modified to minimize skill and competition and maximize participant enjoyment. As a result, smiles and laughter often replace the grunting and groaning that are associated with more traditional exercise programs.

This comprehensive listing of activity (exercise) ideas should prove to be a useful and unique reference to fitness instructors, exercise leaders, aerobics teachers, physiologists, physical educators, therapists, and researchers who are interested in stimulating and maintaining interest, enthusiasm, and adherence among program participants.

iv

The first chapter provides an overview of the exercise compliance problem and the potential variables contributing to it. Chapters 2 through 5 review the keys to a successful adult fitness or cardiac exercise program, with specific reference to safety, effectiveness, education/motivation strategies, and a fun or pleasure principle. The remaining chapters provide hundreds of pleasurable exercises that are clearly illustrated, including individual and partner stationary and continuous movement activities, group activities, recreational games and relays, and special stunts designed to challenge balance, flexibility, and coordination.

Our acknowledgements begin with Brenda White who meticulously coordinated the word processing and editing of this book with a unique sense of pride, perfection, and perseverance. Special thanks also go to Patricia Banks, an extraordinarily talented graphic artist, for the detailed drawings and figures that she prepared for several of the chapters, and to Pete Roberts, for his photographic contributions. We would also like to express appreciation to William Loechel, a medical illustrator par excellence, who captured our exercise ideas on paper with his artistic wizardry. Furthermore, we would like to express our gratitude to Irving (Butch) Cooper and Kendal Gladish, our publisher and editor, respectively, for their patience, encouragement, and expertise.

Finally, we would like to thank our many past and present exercise program participants who served as experimental subjects for the activities presented in this book. Over the years they have tested each of these activities in our exercise laboratory — the gymnasium. Many of our ideas (or dreams) were well-received; others (nightmares) bombed. Those receiving a "thumbs up" are presented here.

Barry A. Franklin, Ph.D.
Neil B. Oldridge, Ph.D.
Karl G. Stoedefalke, Ph.D.

1

Maximizing Compliance

Although numerous variables are related to and predictive of the exercise dropout (Table 1-1),[13] *the exercise leader appears to be the single most important variable affecting exercise compliance.*[10,21,26] Knowledgeable and trained exercise leaders play a critical role in the development and implementation of adult fitness and cardiac exercise programs. Additionally, they are responsible for: (a) educating participants *why* and *how* they should be physically active, and (b) motivating them to follow through with personal exercise programs.[23,26,30]

This book was written for the exercise leader or fitness program director who is interested in stimulating and maintaining interest, enthusiasm, and adherence among program participants. It reviews the keys to a successful adult fitness or cardiac exercise program, highlighting the "Games-As-Aerobics" ap-

TABLE 1-1. Variables Predicting the Exercise Dropout*

Personal factors
1. Smoker
2. Inactive leisure time
3. Inactive occupation
4. Blue collar worker
5. Type A personality
6. Increased physical strength
7. Extroverted
8. Poor credit rating
9. Overweight and/or low ponderal index
10. Poor self-motivation
11. Depressed
12. Hypochondriacal
13. Anxious
14. Introverted
15. Low ego strength

Program factors
1. Inconvenient time/location
2. Excessive cost
3. High intensity exercise
4. Lack of exercise variety, e.g., running only
5. Exercises alone
6. Lack of positive feedback or reinforcement
7. Inflexible exercise goals
8. Low enjoyment ratings for running programs
9. Poor exercise leadership

Other factors
1. Lack of spouse support
2. Inclement weather
3. Excessive job travel
4. Injury
5. Job change/move

*Adapted from Franklin, B.A.[13]

proach to physical activity as well as the importance of four specific objectives:

- To Maintain Safety
- To Promote Effectiveness
- To Emphasize Educational/Motivational Strategies
- To Encourage the Fun or Pleasure Principle

EXERCISE COMPLIANCE

Exercise training is widely advocated in the prevention and treatment of several "chronic" health problems. Appropriately prescribed endurance exercise training, when maintained on a regular basis, has a favorable effect on cardiorespiratory function and maximal oxygen consumption ($\dot{V}O_2$max).[7] Aerobic exercise training programs can result in moderate losses in body weight, moderate-to-large losses in body fat, and small-to-moderate increases in lean body weight.[31] Regular endurance exercise can also promote decreases in blood pressure (particularly among hypertensives), serum triglycerides, and low-density lipoprotein cholesterol and increases in the "antiatherogenic" high-density lipoprotein cholesterol subfraction.[4],[28] Unfortunately, conventional exercise programs are often ineffective in achieving these outcomes, with poor participant compliance a big part of the problem. [12],[27]

Adult fitness and cardiac exercise programs have typically reported dropout rates ranging from 9 to 87 percent ($\bar{x}$ = 44 to 46 percent), highlighting the compliance problem among those who voluntarily enter physical conditioning programs (Figure 1-1).[14],[26] Although widely differing definitions of "exercise dropout" in these studies may have contributed to the variability in results, it appears that exercise is not unlike other health-related behaviors (e.g., medication compliance, smoking cessation, weight reduction) in that *typically half or less of those who initiate the behavior will continue,* irrespective of initial health status or type of program.

The traditional approach to the exercise compliance problem has involved attempting to persuade dropouts to become reinvolved. An alternative approach, however, would involve the identification and subsequent monitoring of "dropout prone" individuals, with an aim toward preventing recidivism.[13] Accordingly, it would be necessary to characterize individuals in terms of exercise dropout proneness, an area of considerable research over the past 20 years.

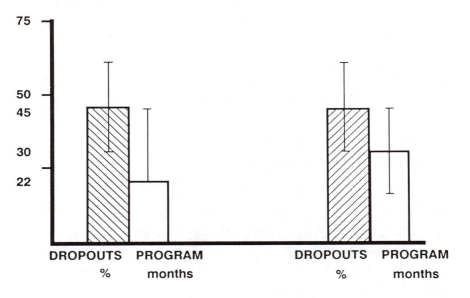

Figure 1-1. Relationship between the dropout rate (%) and the duration of exercise training (months) in 8 studies with a total of 525 healthy adults and 12 studies with a total of 3,085 cardiac patients.[14],[26]

Exercise Dropout

Principal factors related to long-term exercise noncompliance include cigarette smoking, blue collar employment, inactive leisure time, and inactive occupation; others are listed in Table 1-1. The noncompliance rate appears to increase progressively, from 59 percent in the presence of smoking alone, the single most discriminating variable, to 95 percent with all four variables.[23],[25] Additional characteristics predictive of the exercise dropout may include overweight,[1],[20] a poor credit rating,[15] Type A personality,[22] and increased physical strength.[20] Psychological traits that predict noncompliance to exercise include depression, hypochondriasis, anxiety, marked introversion or extroversion,[20] and low ego strength.[3] Although morbid obesity has generally been associated with poor exercise compliance,[5] our experience with a 12-week exercise training program,[11] and an 18-month follow-up investigation,[16] revealed no difference in initial adherence or maintenance of the exercise habit among lean to normal weight and moderately obese middle-aged women.

Exercise program variables such as inconvenient location,[29] excessive cost, and higher intensity training,[17] with its disproportionate incidence of orthopedic injuries, have been associated with lower compliance rates. Lack of social reinforcement during exercise, specifically individual as opposed to group participation, has also been related to poor adherence.[15],[20] Other factors recently found to predict nonadherence include extreme weather conditions, goal inflexibility, and lower enjoyment ratings for programs that emphasize running alone.[18],[19]

Self-motivation levels,[8] contracting and self-monitoring[24],[25] as well as goal-setting[6] also appear to influence exercise compliance. A brief questionnaire[8],[9] designed to assess "self-motivation" showed mixed accuracy when predicting male and female exercise dropout-prone behavior (Table 1-2). When combined with measures of total body weight and percent body fat, the self-motivation scores were found to accurately classify participants according to their adherence status in approximately 80 percent of all cases.[8],[9] Finally, individuals who fail to attain their personal exercise goals demonstrate approximately twice the dropout rate as those who do attain them.[6]

Reasons Why Individuals Discontinue Exercise Training

Data from the Ontario Exercise-Heart Collaborative Study revealed that 42 percent of the "dropouts" discontinued exercise

TABLE 1-2. Self-Motivation Assessment Scale to Determine Likelihood of Exercise Compliance[a]

A	B	C	D	E	
5	4	3	2	1	1. I get discouraged easily.
5	4	3	2	1	2. I don't work any harder than I have to.
1	2	3	4	5	3. I seldom if ever let myself down.
5	4	3	2	1	4. I'm just not the goal-setting type.
1	2	3	4	5	5. I'm good at keeping promises, especially the ones I make to myself.
5	4	3	2	1	6. I don't impose much structure on my activities.
1	2	3	4	5	7. I have a very hard-driving, aggressive personality.

Directions: Circle the number beneath the letter corresponding to the alternative that best describes how characteristic the statement is when applied to you. The alternatives are:

    A.   *extremely* uncharacteristic of me.
    B.   *somewhat* uncharacteristic of me.
    C.   neither characteristic nor uncharacteristic of me.
    D.   *somewhat* characteristic of me.
    E.   *extremely* characteristic of me.

Scoring: Add together the seven numbers you circled. A score equal to or less than *24* suggests dropout-prone behavior. The lower the self-motivation score, the greater the likelihood toward exercise noncompliance. If the score suggests dropout proneness, it should be viewed as an incentive to remain active, rather than a self-fulfilling prophecy to quit exercising.

[a]Copyright 1978 by R.K. Dishman and W.J. Ickes. From Falls, H.B. et al.[9]
Reproduced by permission of the copyright holders.

for psychosocial reasons, including lack of interest, poor motivation, and/or family problems; 25 percent for unavoidable reasons such as job shift or residence change; 22 percent for medical reasons, some associated with inappropriate exercise programming; and 11 percent for other reasons.[22] Thus, psychosocial variables, including perception of the program, personal convenience factors, and family lifestyle components appear to present the major impediment to exercise compliance, accounting for almost half of the dropouts.[22,26]

    Compared to compliers, noncompliers generally lacked enthusiasm for the program and frequently reported post-exercise fatigue. Similarly, dropouts found it more difficult to arrive on time for the exercise programs; their jobs were perceived to interfere more with attendance.[1,2] Those who found it difficult to relax after work, and those whose incomes had not reached their expectations, also had significantly lower compliance rates.[1,2] Participants with spouses who were neutral or negative regarding their exercise habits were also only half as likely to have excellent or good adherence as compared with those whose spouses were positive toward the program.[2,15]

BIBLIOGRAPHY

1. Andrew, G.M. and J.O. Parker. (1979) "Factors Related to Dropout of Post Myocardial Infarction Patients From Exercise Programs." *Med. Sci. Sports,* 11:376–378.
2. Andrew, G.M., N.B. Oldridge, J.O. Parker, et al. (1981) "Reasons for Dropout from Exercise Programs in Post-Coronary Patients." *Med. Sci. Sports Exerc.,* 13:164–168.
3. Blumenthal, J.A., R.S. Williams, A.G. Wallace, et al. (1982) "Physiological and Psychological Variables Predict Compliance to Prescribed Exercise Therapy in Patients Recovering from Myocardial Infarction." *Psychosom. Med.,* 44:519–527.
4. Boyer, J.L. and F.W. Kasch. (1970) "Exercise Therapy in Hypertensive Men." *J.A.M.A.,* 211:1668–1671.
5. Buskirk, E.R. (1974) "Obesity: A Brief Overview With Emphasis on Exercise." *Fed. Proc.,* 33:1948–1951.
6. Danielson, R.R. and R.S. Wanzel. (1978) "Exercise Objectives of Fitness Program Dropouts." In Landers, D.M. and R.W. Christina (eds.): *Psychology of Motor Behavior and Sports.* Champaign, Illinois, Human Kinetics Publishers.
7. Davis, J., M. Frank, B. Whipp, et al. (1979) "Anaerobic Threshold Alterations Caused by Endurance Training in Middle-Aged Men." *J. Appl. Physiol.,* 46:1039–1046.
8. Dishman, R.K., W. Ickes and W.P. Morgan. (1980) "Self-Motivation and Adherence to Habitual Physical Activity." *J. Appl. Social Psychol.,* 10:115–132.
9. Falls, H.B., A.M. Baylor and R.K. Dishman. (1980) *Essentials of Fitness.* Appendix A-13. Philadelphia, Saunders College.
10. Franklin, B. "Motivating and Educating Adults to Exercise." (1978) *J. Phys. Ed. Rec.,* 49:13–17.
11. Franklin, B., E. Buskirk, J. Hodgson, et al. (1979) "Effects of Physical Conditioning on Cardiorespiratory Function, Body Composition and Serum Lipids in Relatively Normal-Weight and Obese Middle-Aged Women." *Intl. J. Obesity,* 3:97–109.
12. Franklin, B. and M. Rubenfire. (1980) "Losing Weight Through Exercise." *J.A.M.A.,* 244:377–379.
13. Franklin, B.A. (1984) "Exercise Program Compliance: Improvement Strategies." In Storlie, J. and H.A. Jordan (eds.): *Behavioral Management of Obesity.* New York, Spectrum Publications, Inc., pp. 105–135.
14. Franklin, B.A. (1988) "Program Factors That Influence Exercise Adherence: Practical Adherence Skills for the Clinical Staff." In Dishman, R. (ed.): *Exercise Adherence: Its Impact on Public Health.* Champaign, Human Kinetics, pp. 237–258.
15. Heinzelman, F. and R.W. Bagley. (1970) "Response to Physical Activity Programs and Their Effects on Health Behavior." *Public Health Rep.,* 85:905–911.
16. MacKeen, P.C., B.A. Franklin, W.C. Nicholas, et al. (1983) "Body Composition, Physical Work Capacity and Physical Activity Habits at Eighteen-Month Follow-Up of Middle-Aged Women Participating in an Exercise Intervention." *Intl. J. Obesity,* 7:61–71.
17. Mann, G.V., H.L. Garrett, A. Farhi, et al. (1969) "Exercise to Prevent Coronary Heart Disease: An Experimental Study of the Effects of Training on Risk Factors for Coronary Disease in Men." *Am. J. Med.,* 46:12–27.
18. Martin, J.E. (1981) "Exercise Management: Shaping and Maintaining Physical Fitness." *Behav. Med. Advances,* 4:3–5.
19. Martin, J.E. and P.M. Dubbert. (1982) "Exercise Applications and Promotion in Behavioral Medicine: Current Status and Future Directions." *J. Consult. Clin. Psychol.,* 50:1004–1017.
20. Massie, J.F. and R.J. Shephard. (1971) "Physiological and Psychological Effects of Training — A Comparison of Individual and Gymnasium Programs, With a Characterization of the Exercise 'Drop-Out'." *Med. Sci. Sports,* 3:110–117.
21. Oldridge, N. (1977) "What to Look For in an Exercise Class Leader." *Phys. Sportsmed.,* 5:85–88.

22. Oldridge, N.B., J.R. Wicks, C. Hanley, et al. (1978) "Noncompliance in an Exercise Rehabilitation Program for Men Who Have Suffered a Myocardial Infarction," *Can. Med. Assoc., J.*, 118:361–364.
23. Oldridge, N.B., A.P. Donner, C.W. Buck, et al. (1983) "Predictors of Dropout from Cardiac Rehabilitation. Ontario Exercise Heart Collaborative Study." *Am. J. Cardiol.*, 51:70–74.
24. Oldridge, N.B. and N.L. Jones. (1983) "Improving Patient Compliance in Cardiac Exercise Rehabilitation: Effects of Written Agreement and Self-Monitoring." *J. Cardiac Rehabil.* 3:257–262.
25. Oldridge, N.B. and N.L. Jones. (1986) "Preventive Use of Exercise Rehabilitation after Myocardial Infarction." *Acta Med. Scand.*, Suppl. 711:123–129.
26. Oldridge, N.B. (1988) "Compliance with Exercise Rehabilitation." In Dishman, R. (ed.): *Exercise Adherence: Its Impact on Public Health*. Champaign, Illinois, Human Kinetics, pp. 283–304.
27. Rejewski, W.J. and E.A. Kenney. (1988) *Fitness Motivation: Preventing Participant Dropout.* Champaign, Illinois, Life Enhancement Publications.
28. Streja, D. and D. Mymin. (1979) "Moderate Exercise and High Density Lipoprotein Cholesterol: Observations During a Cardiac Rehabilitation Program." *J.A.M.A.*, 242:2190–2192.
29. Teraslinna, P., T. Partanen, A. Koskela, et al. (1969) "Characteristics Affecting Willingness of Executives to Participate in an Activity Program Aimed at Coronary Heart Disease Prevention." *J. Sports Med. Phys.* Fitness, 9:224–229.
30. Wilmore, J.H. (1974) "Individual Exercise Prescription." *Am. J. Cardiol.*, 33:757–759.
31. Wilmore, J. (1983) "Body Composition in Sport and Exercise: Directions for Future Research." *Med. Sci. Sports*, 15:21–31.

2

Maximizing Program Safety

The safety of an adult fitness program depends, to a large extent, on five factors: selection of appropriate exercises and equipment, competent exercise leaders, established injury/emergency plans, careful preliminary testing and follow-up of participants, and coping with environmental conditions such as weather extremes.[5]

SELECTION OF APPROPRIATE EXERCISES AND EQUIPMENT

Previously sedentary adults often have unrealistic impressions of safe and effective exercise practices. The exercise leader should select activities that limit the potential for musculoskeletal and orthopedic complications, yet meet a minimum exercise dosage (frequency, intensity, duration) that will increase cardiorespiratory fitness and promote a negative caloric balance.[17] Excessive fatigue, extreme muscle soreness, and injury must be avoided if such regimens are to be maintained. The challenge is to recognize what constitutes an overload for deconditioned adults and to be enthusiastic about achievements that may seem insignificant. Activity leaders must forgo the temptation to impose exercise programs suitable for the leaders' physical conditioning and skills rather than the participants'.

Probably the most appropriate warm-up activity is the actual activity to be carried out, but at a lower intensity; brisk walking before slow jogging, jogging before running. Although calisthenics are generally recommended before vigorous endurance activity, adults should not perform deep knee bends, full squats, squat jumps, duck-walk movements, and other exercises that force the knee joint into full flexion.[19] Ligament complications, cartilage tears, and relaxation of the knee joint may result. Leg lifts have also been criticized because of the potential for low back injury. Sit-ups or push-ups, if employed, should be performed with the legs flexed at the knee joint. Simply lifting the shoulder blades off the ground constitutes an effective sit-up in the initial stages of an exercise program.

In recent years "miracle exercise devices" and special weight reducing garments have been touted to the gullible consumer.[6] These include motor-driven bicycles, electrical stimulating devices, mechanical vibrators/rollers, waist trimming and vibrator belts, and rubberized sweat suits.[7] Although clever advertisers suggest that fitness or weight loss can be achieved "without vigorous exercise," there are no data to substantiate these claims. Moreover, some of these gadgets and gimmicks may be hazardous. Rubberized sweat suits, for example, actually prevent the evaporation of sweat, depriving the body of its normal cooling mechanism. Exercise-related heat disorders may result, such as heat cramps, heat exhaustion, or heat stroke.

COMPETENT EXERCISE LEADERS

Knowledgeable and trained exercise leaders play an essential role in exercise program safety.[14] Program personnel should realize that the muscles, joints, and ligaments of previously sedentary adults are not accustomed to sudden strenuous movements. Fitness instructors need to consider the preventive value of warm-up and cool-down, the misinformation that pervades the field of fitness (e.g., never drink while exercising, use salt tablets in the heat), the importance of appropriate clothing and shoes, the influence of heat and/or humidity on performance, and the signs and symptoms of overexertion, as well as appropriate remedial actions.[23]

Exercise instructors should have training and experience leading workshops or teaching in a group setting. Evidence of continuing education through the American College of Sports Medicine (ACSM) or other certifications is desirable, with training and regular practice in first aid and basic cardiopulmonary resuscitation (CPR).

ESTABLISHED INJURY/ EMERGENCY PROCEDURES

Adult fitness and cardiac exercise programs should establish policies and procedures regarding the on-site treatment of musculoskeletal complications and emergency situations.[5] First aid supplies, ice, and fruit juice should be readily available; for example, a diabetic client who may occasionally become hypoglycemic (low blood sugar) during or after a workout can benefit from fruit juice. Exercise leaders should also be prepared to handle the rare instance of a cardiovascular complication.[13,21] This includes performing basic CPR and stabilizing the participant for transport to an emergency medical center. To this end, emergency drills should be conducted regularly, and a plan of action should be established in which specific responsibilities are assigned (e.g., perform CPR, call emergency medical services, clear participants from the immediate area, wait for and direct the emergency medical team to the victim.) Finally, numbers for emergency medical assistance should be clearly labeled on all telephones.

PRELIMINARY SCREENING/ FOLLOW-UP TESTING

According to the ACSM guidelines:

". . . exercise is a safe activity for most individuals. However, it is desirable for adults to have some screening prior to starting an exercise program or taking an exercise test. It has become apparent that for many individuals the pre-exercise evaluation can be done by nonmedical personnel in nonmedical settings. Age, health status, type of test, and exercise plan are factors which determine the depth of evaluation required and the need for medical involvement."[2]

The first task of exercise leaders and/or program directors is to learn something about the people they intend to serve. Many programs recommend that participants complete a battery of fitness and laboratory tests prior to starting an exercise regimen. However, privacy and a pleasant physical setting are essential when clients are evaluated and interviewed. Evaluations may include: a self-administered medical history form (Table 2-1); health lifestyle questionnaire; hydrostatic weighing[1] or subcutaneous skinfold thickness measurements for assessment of percent body fatness and ideal weight; standard spirometry (e.g., vital capacity, $FEV_{1.0}$ and FEF_{25-75}); flexibility testing (e.g., sit-and-reach test);[10] grip strength evaluation; and a

TABLE 2-1. Self-administered Pre-Exercise Medical History

Name _____ Weight _____ Height_____

Please check all boxes which pertain to you:

PERSONAL HISTORY — PAST	PRESENT	FAMILY HISTORY
		Have any of your relatives ever had:
1. ☐ Rheumatic fever	11. ☐ Chest pain	18. ☐ Heart attacks
2. ☐ Heart murmur	12. ☐ Shortness of breath	19. ☐ High blood pressure
3. ☐ High blood pressure	13. ☐ Heart palpitations	20. ☐ Too much cholesterol
4. ☐ Any heart trouble	14. ☐ Cough on exertion	21. ☐ Diabetes
5. ☐ Disease of arteries	15. ☐ Back pain	22. ☐ Congenital heart disease
6. ☐ Varicose veins	.16. ☐ Swollen, stiff or painful joints	23. ☐ Heart operations
7. ☐ Lung disease	17. ☐ Dizziness	24. ☐ Stroke
8. ☐ Heart operations		25. ☐ Other (specify):
9. ☐ Injuries to back, etc.		
10. ☐ Diabetes		

COMMENTS _____
_____
_____
_____
_____
_____
_____
_____
_____
_____

PERSONAL HABITS

1. Smoking:
   Cigarettes: ☐ Yes ☐ No ☐ Quit   Date _____ How many/day_____ Duration (years) _____
   Cigars: ☐ Yes ☐ No ☐ Quit   Date _____ How many/day_____ Duration (years) _____
   Pipe: ☐ Yes ☐ No ☐ Quit   Date _____ How many/day_____ Duration (years) _____

2. Alcohol Consumption: ☐ Yes ☐ No   How much _____ oz./week

3. Body Weight:
   What is your weight now? _____ 1 year ago _____ at age 21 _____
   Are you dieting? ☐ Yes ☐ No

4. Is your occupation: ☐ Sedentary (desk work)   ☐ Active (some walking)   ☐ Very active (walking constantly)   ☐ Heavy work (labor)

5. Exercise Program _____   Intensity _____

   Frequency _____   Duration _____

12- to 14-hour fasting serum lipid and lipoprotein profile (e.g., total cholesterol, triglycerides, HDL-cholesterol). Simple screening measures such as height, weight, and waist or hip girth can also be used to estimate relative body fatness in men and women (Figure 2-1).[22]

Exercise tolerance testing may be recommended for several reasons: 1) to aid in the diagnosis of hidden or latent coronary heart disease in asymptomatic or symptomatic individuals (Figure 2-2); 2) to evaluate cardiopulmonary fitness; 3) to establish the safety of vigorous exercise prior to initiating a physical conditioning program[3,11]; and 4) to assess work-related capabilities. Recently, however, the need for exercise testing as a screening procedure in asymptomatic adults who exercise in recreation facilities has been questioned.[18] Critics emphasize that the cost of mass screenings would be prohibitive. Furthermore, the incidence of exercise-related cardiovascular complications in presumably healthy adults is extremely low.[13,21] These findings, in addition to the uncertainties associated with exercise-induced ST-segment depression in persons with a low pre-test likelihood of coronary heart disease,[8] would suggest

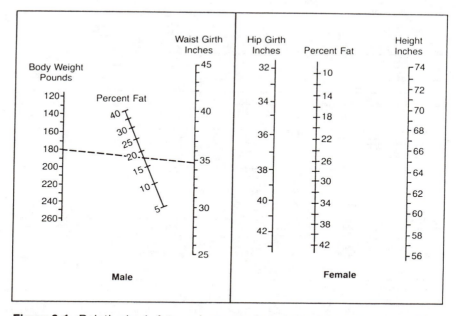

Figure 2-1. Relative body fatness in men and women can be estimated (± 10%) with a simple tape measure and a straight edge, using these charts. For example, a 180-pound male with a 34¾-inch waist would have an estimated relative fatness of 18%. Applying the margin of error will yield a body fat range of 16.2% to 19.8%. Adapted from Wilmore, J.H.[22]

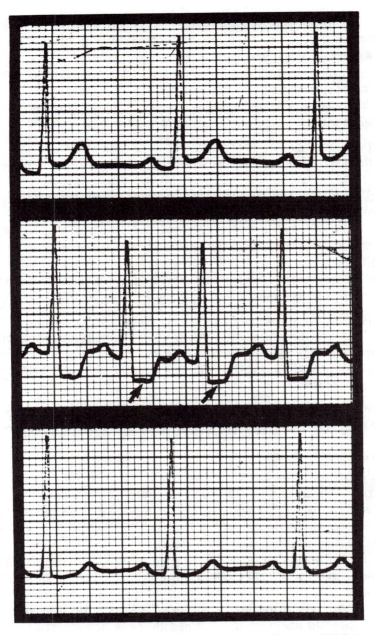

Figure 2-2. (Top) An individual's resting electrocardiogram (ECG; lead V5) taken before exercise testing. (Middle) ECG obtained after several minutes of an exercise test. Inadequate blood supply to the heart muscle caused a characteristic change in the ECG pattern called ST-segment depression (arrow). (Bottom) Resting ECG recorded 6 minutes after exercise. It is again representative of a "normal" ECG.

that it is impractical to use routine exercise testing to prevent significant cardiovascular complications among adults who initiate exercise programs.[20]

In summary, the need for exercise testing of asymptomatic physically active people remains a controversial issue. Guidelines from the ACSM recommend maximal exercise tests for the following individuals starting an exercise program:[2]

- Apparently healthy individuals at or above age 45.
- Individuals at or above age 35 with at least one of the following coronary risk factors: history of high blood pressure (above 145/95 mmHg); elevated total cholesterol/high-density lipoprotein cholesterol ratio (above 5); cigarette smoking; abnormal resting electrocardiogram; family history of coronary or other atherosclerotic disease prior to age 50; and diabetes mellitus.
- Individuals at any age with known cardiovascular, pulmonary, or metabolic disease.

These recommendations are in contrast to earlier ACSM guidelines, which suggested maximal exercise tests for inactive, asymptomatic persons 35 years of age or older without coronary risk factors, and asymptomatic persons of any age with coronary risk factors.[4]

COPING WITH ENVIRONMENTAL CONDITIONS
Warm Weather

Vigorous exercise when the environmental temperature or humidity is high can lead to heat stress. Such stress places excessive demands on the circulation and other body mechanisms that attempt to dissipate heat generated by the environment and the increased metabolism of exercise.

The body has a marvelous thermostat to prevent dramatic increases in temperature. A substantial portion of the blood flow is diverted from the core or center of the body to the surface (skin) where it is more easily cooled. This is the reason underlying the flushed appearance of the skin on a hot summer day.

In addition, evaporation of sweat on the skin serves as a powerful mechanism to cool the body. Remember: *It is not sweating that cools the body, rather the evaporation of sweat into the atmosphere.*

Malfunctions in the temperature regulation mechanism can result from excessive body water losses or high humidity. Both can decrease the effectiveness of the sweating response. Excessive water losses reduce the magnitude of sweating. With high humidity, very little sweat is actually absorbed by the surrounding moisture-laden air, and the sweat merely rolls off the body. As a result, body heat tends to increase abruptly, driving core temperature upward. Heat stroke and related complications may occur.

Several suggestions are offered to help reduce heat stress when working or exercising in hot and/or humid environments:

- Maintain salt-water balance by drinking plenty of cool fluids (either water or a weak salt solution) before, during, and after physical activity.
- Exercise during the cooler parts of the day, preferably when the sun's radiation is minimal (early morning or early evening).
- Decrease exercise intensity and duration at high temperatures and/or relative humidity (Table 2-2). Under such conditions, a reduced walking or jogging speed or power output will achieve the recommended training heart rate.[15]
- Wear minimal amounts of clothing to facilitate cooling by evaporation. Porous, light-colored, cotton clothing is ideal. Rubberized sweat suits, often worn to "enhance weight loss," block sweat losses by evaporation and thus deprive the body of its normal mechanism for cooling. Severe heat stress may result.
- Allow the body to adapt partially to heat through repeated gradual daily exposures. An increase in the body's circulatory and cooling efficiency (called acclimatization) generally occurs in only 4 to 14 days.[12] Following this brief period, the body is far better able to cope with extremes in heat and humidity.

TABLE 2-2. Heat Stress Index: Exercise Recommendations

% Relative humidity	Temperature								
	60	65	70	75	80	85	90	95	100
0									
10	59	62	64	67	69	72	74	77	79
20	59	62	65	68	70	73	76	79	82
30	59	62	65	68	72	75	78	81	84
40	59	63	66	69	73	76	79	83	86
50	59	63	67	70	74	76	81	85	88
60	60	63	67	71	75	79	83	87	91
70	60	64	68	72	76	81	85	88	93
80	60	64	69	73	78	82	86	91	95
90	60	65	69	74	79	84	88	93	98
100	60	65	70	75	80	85	90	95	100
			Caution		*Extreme caution*				

Cold Weather

Outdoor exercise during the winter months usually presents fewer problems than expected. Adequate clothing promotes heat conservation while exercise actually serves as an "antidote" to cold, increasing body heat production.

Physiologically, the body acts to conserve its own heat by reducing blood flow to the skin (vasoconstriction). Thus, heat is conserved within its vital inner regions. If this first line of defense is inadequate, the body shivers, which adds to the metabolic heat production.

A few extra precautions will help prevent excessive exposure to cold:[9]

- Be extra careful when the wind is blowing. Temperature alone is not a valid index of cold stress. The wind removes the layer of air that the body has heated around it to keep it warm. The "wind chill factor" measures the effective decrease in temperature resulting from moving air. For example, at 10 degrees Fahrenheit in a 20-mile-an-hour wind, the cooling effect is equivalent to calm air at minus 25 degrees (Table 2-3).
- Beware of wet clothing. Since water is an excellent conductor, damp clothing presents a problem because it extracts heat from the body much faster than dry clothing. For this reason, adults should be encouraged to change wet clothing, particularly socks and gloves.
- Dress appropriately. Overdressing for exercise in the cold may result in overheating and excessive sweating. *A handy rule for dressing for exercise in the cold is to wear several*

TABLE 2-3. Effects of Wind and Low Temperature

WIND CHILL FACTOR TABLE

Estimated wind speed (in mph)	Actual thermometer reading (in degrees Fahrenheit)					
	30°	20°	10°	0°	-10°	-20°
	EQUIVALENT TEMPERATURE					
Calm	30	20	10	0	-10	-20
10	16	4	-9	-24	-33	-46
20	4	-10	-25	-39	-53	-67
30	-2	-18	-33	-48	-63	-78
40	-6	-21	-37	-53	-69	-86

*Adapted from Pollock, M.L. et al.[16]

layers of light clothing that can be shed or replaced separately as body heat changes. Between each layer, there is trapped air which, when heated by the body, acts as an excellent insulator.

The insulating properties of wool are widely recognized. It is one material which, when wet, still keeps the body warm. Most other materials, when wet, actually draw heat from the body and pass it into the air.

- Stay moving. Because of the potential 10- to 20-fold increase in heat production during strenuous exercise, body temperature can be easily maintained even in subzero conditions, as long as one continues to exercise. Outdoor exercisers should avoid standing still for too long in the cold. They should move their arms and legs, walk, or jog in place to get the large muscles working.

- Protect certain body areas. Body heat is most easily lost from parts that have a large surface area to mass ratio — for example, the hands and feet. Keep them warm and dry. Mittens, or gloves under mittens, are preferable to gloves alone. For the feet, two pairs of wool socks are ideal. Because of a poor vasoconstriction response, a tremendous loss of body heat (at least 25 percent) can occur from an uncovered head. Always wear a hat or cap when exercising in the cold.

BIBLIOGRAPHY

1. Akers, R. and E.R. Buskirk. (1969) "An Underwater Weighing System Utilizing 'Force Cube' Transducers." *J. Appl. Physiol.*, 26:649-652.
2. American College of Sports Medicine. (1986) *Guidelines for Graded Exercise Testing and Exercise Prescription*. 3rd ed., Philadelphia: Lea and Febiger.
3. *American College of Sports Medicine Resource Manual for Guidelines for Graded Exercise Testing and Exercise Prescription*. (1988) Blair, S.N., P. Painter, R.R. Pate, L.K. Smith and C.B. Taylor (eds.). Philadelphia: Lea and Febiger.
4. American College of Sports Medicine. (1980) *Guidelines for Graded Exercise Testing and Exercise Prescription*. 2nd ed., Philadelphia: Lea and Febiger.
5. Franklin, B.A. (1986) "Clinical Components of a Successful Adult Fitness Program." *Am. J. Health Promotion*, 1:6-13.
6. Franklin, B. and M. Rubenfire. (1980) "Losing Weight Through Exercise." *J.A.M.A.*, 244:377-379.
7. Franklin, B.A. (1984) "Myths and Misconceptions in Exercise for Weight Control." In Storlie, J. and H.A. Jordan (eds.): *Nutrition and Exercise in Obesity Management*. New York: Spectrum Publications, Inc., pp. 53-92.
8. Franklin, B.A., V. Hollingsworth and L.M. Borysyk. (1988) "Additional Diagnostic Tests: Special Populations." In Blair S.N., P. Painter, R.R. Pate, L.K. Smith and C.B. Taylor (eds): *American College of Sports Resource Manual for Guidelines for Graded Exercise Testing and Exercise Prescription*, Philadelphia, Lea and Febiger, pp. 223-235.
9. Franklin, B.A. (1988) "Take Care in the Cold." *Heartline Bulletin*, 18(12):1-2.
10. Golding, L.A., C.R. Myers and W.E. Sinning (eds.). (1982) *The Y's Way to Physical Fitness*. Chicago: National Board of YMCA.

11. Hellerstein, H.K. and B. Franklin. (1984) "Exercise Testing and Prescription." In Wenger, N.K. and H.K. Hellerstein (eds.): *Rehabilitation of the Coronary Patient.* 2nd ed., New York: John Wiley, pp. 197-284.
12. Lamb, D.R. (1978) *Physiology of Exercise: Responses and Adaptations.* New York: MacMillan.
13. Malinow, M., D. McGarry and K. Kuehl. (1984) "Is Exercise Testing Indicated for Asymptomatic Active People?" *J. Cardiac Rehabil.,* 4:376-380.
14. Oldridge, N. (1977) "What to Look For in an Exercise Class Leader." *Phys. Sportsmed.,* 5:85-88.
15. Pandolf, K.B., E. Cafarelli, B.J. Noble, et al. (1975) "Hyperthermia: Effect on Exercise Prescription." *Arch. Phys. Med. Rehabil.,* 56:524-526.
16. Pollock, M.L., J.H. Wilmore and S.M. Fox (1984). *Exercise in Health and Disease: Evaluation and Prescription for Prevention and Rehabilitation.* Philadelphia: W.B. Saunders Company, p. 384.
17. Rejewski, W.J. and E.A. Kenney. (1988) *Fitness Motivation: Preventing Participant Dropout.* Champaign: Life Enhancement Publications.
18. Solomon, H. (1986) "Undue Exertion: Cardiac Stress Tests Aren't Worth the Money — Or the Risk." *The Sciences,* 12-16, January/February.
19. Stoedefalke, K.G. and J.L. Hodgson. (1975) "Exercise Rx — Designing a Program." *Medical Opinion,* 4:48-55.
20. Thompson, P., E. Funk, R. Carleton, et al. (1982) "Incidence of Death During Jogging in Rhode Island from 1975 through 1980." *J.A.M.A.,* 247:2535-2538.
21. Vander, L., B. Franklin and M. Rubenfire. (1982) "Cardiovascular Complications of Recreational Physical Activity." *Phys. Sportsmed.,* 10:89-98.
22. Wilmore, J. (1986) *Sensible Fitness.* Champaign: Human Kinetics Books.
23. Zohman, L. and A. Kattus. (1979) *The Cardiologist's Guide to Fitness and Health Through Exercise.* New York: Simon and Schuster.

3

Maximizing Program Effectiveness

In addition to sustained compliance, the effectiveness of an exercise program depends on an appropriate exercise prescription. There are three phases to the typical aerobic exercise session: warm-up, endurance phase, and cool-down (Figure 3-1).[28] Recreational games and activities can also be employed after the endurance phase, before the cool-down. A brief review of the physiologic basis and rationale for each phase is provided below.

WARM-UP

The warm-up period, generally lasting 5 to 15 minutes, prepares the body for more intense activity. The goal is to gradually

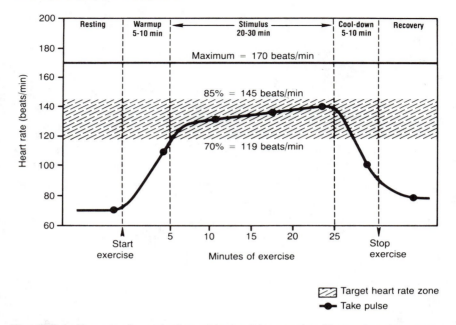

Figure 3-1. Format of a typical aerobic exercise session illustrating the warm-up, stimulus, and cool-down phases along with a representative heart rate response. The target heart rate zone for training corresponds to 70 to 85 percent of the peak heart rate achieved during maximal exercise testing. (Adapted from Zohman, L.R.)[28]

raise the participant's metabolic rate to an acceptable target level. The warm-up serves as a period of adaptation by increasing blood flow and enhancing the efficiency of working muscle.[26] Moreover, a preliminary warm-up serves to decrease the susceptibility to injury and the occurrence of electrocardiographic abnormalities that are suggestive of myocardial ischemia and/or ventricular irritability — abnormalities that may be provoked by sudden strenuous exertion.[3,4,5,12] Thus, warm-up has preventive value and enhances performance capacity.[18]

Warm-up exercises should include both musculoskeletal (i.e., stretching, flexibility, and muscle-strengthening exercises) and cardiorespiratory activities. Although exercise physiologists have presented a strong case for the superiority of static over ballistic stretching techniques, the latter can still improve flexibility. An initial period of calisthenics, involving stretching and flexibility movements, may include flexion, extension, circling, rotation, abduction, and adduction. A cardiorespiratory warm-up should follow and involve total body movement to include an intensity of activity (i.e., alternate walking-jogging, swimming-recovering, mild-moderate cycling) sufficient to evoke a heart rate response within 20 beats/minute of the heart rate recommended for endurance training.

Our experience suggests that the ideal warm-up for any endurance activity is that activity only at a lower intensity.[14] Hence, participants who use brisk walking during the endurance phase should conclude the warm-up period with slow walking. Similarly, brisk walking (i.e., 3.5 to 4.5 mph) serves as an ideal warm-up for participants who jog during the endurance phase. Cardiorespiratory warm-up activities can also be modified to incorporate playground balls and individual, partner, or group activities or relays. However, with partner or small group activities, participants should be grouped with individuals who have similar aerobic capacities ($\dot{V}O_2$max).

ENDURANCE OR STIMULUS PHASE

The endurance phase (at least 20 to 30 minutes) serves to directly stimulate the oxygen transport system and maximize caloric expenditure. This phase should be prescribed in specific terms of intensity (how strenuously a person exercises), frequency (how often a person exercises), duration (how long is each exercise session), and mode (the type of exercise that is best). Using an "Exercise Prescription Form" (Table 3-1) provides an ideal way of ensuring your recommendations to the participant. It should be emphasized, however, that interrelationships among these variables may permit a sub-threshold level in one factor to be partially or totally compensated for by appropriate increases in one or both of the others.[1]

Exercise intensity may be regulated by several popular methods: *a prescribed training heart rate range; assigned pace for walking or jogging; recommended workload for the stationary cycle ergometer; and the Borg category or category-ratio scales for rating of perceived exertion.*[8] This latter method, particularly when used in conjunction with other clinical, psychological, and physiological information (i.e., pulse rate), provides a reliable method for regulating exercise intensity within safe and effective limits.

The Borg perceived exertion scale consists of 15 grades from 6 to 20 or 10 grades from 0 to 10+ (Figure 3-2).[8] The ratings, based on one's overall feeling of exertion and physical fatigue, correspond quite well with metabolic changes (e.g., heart rate, oxygen consumption) experienced during exercise. Participants are cautioned not to overemphasize any one factor, such as leg pain or shortness of breath, but to try to assess their total,

TABLE 3-1. Exercise Prescription Form

M.D. _____

EXERCISE PRESCRIPTION

Name _____ Age _____ Starting Date _____

Clinical Status:

Arrhythmia   Angina   CABG   CAD   HTN   MI   Normal   VR

NOTE: **This prescription is valid only if you remain on the same medications (type and dose),** and you are in the same clinical status as on the day your exercise test was conducted.

CONTRAINDICATIONS: *Angina at rest   *Fever   *Illness
*Temperature and Weather Extremes (below 30 degrees or over 80 degrees with high humidity)

ACTIVITIES TO AVOID: *Sudden strenuous lifting or carrying
*Exertion that leads to holding your breath

EXERCISE TYPE: Aerobic types of exercise that are continuous, dynamic and repetitive in nature

FREQUENCY: _____ times/day _____ days/week

DURATION: Total duration of exercise session: _____ minutes

TO BE DIVIDED AS FOLLOWS:

WARM-UP: (light flexibility/stretching routine) _____ minutes

AEROBIC TRAINING ACTIVITY: _____ to _____ minutes

COOL DOWN: (slow walking and stretching):_____ minutes

INTENSITY:

TARGET HEART RATE _____ to _____ beats/minute

_____ to _____ beats/10 seconds

PERCEIVED EXERTION SHOULD NOT EXCEED "SOMEWHAT HARD"

REEVALUATION

Your next graded exercise test is due: _____

Call our office to schedule an appointment.   Phone **288-7243**

Exercise Physiologist_____

inner feelings of exertion. Among healthy young persons, the effort rating on the 6 to 20 scale generally approximates one-tenth of the heart rate response.

Although the Borg scale provides a useful adjunct to heart rate as the exercise intensity monitor, reflecting a natural and individualized integration of information, the exercise leader should recognize its potential limitations, particularly in novice exercisers and extreme "Type A" individuals. It is doubtful that

PERCEIVED EXERTION

Category Scale

6	
7	VERY, VERY LIGHT
8	
9	VERY LIGHT
10	
11	FAIRLY LIGHT
12	
13	SOMEWHAT HARD
14	
15	HARD
16	
17	VERY HARD
18	
19	VERY, VERY, HARD
20	

Category - ratio Scale

0	NOTHING AT ALL	
0.5	VERY, VERY WEAK	[just noticeable]
1	VERY WEAK	
2	WEAK	[light]
3	MODERATE	
4	SOMEWHAT STRONG	
5	STRONG	[heavy]
6		
7	VERY STRONG	
8		
9		
10	VERY, VERY STRONG	[almost max]
	MAXIMAL	

Figure 3-2. Perceived exertion scales with descriptive "effort ratings." (From Borg, G.)[8]

the former have the experience to regulate work intensity primarily by subjective perceptions, whereas the latter, who are achievement-oriented, compulsive, and highly competitive, have a tendency to deny or ignore physical symptoms. As a result, Type A individuals are often at or above the upper limits of their prescribed heart rate ranges, at relatively low ratings of perceived exertion.

Exercise rated as 11 to 13 (6-20 scale) or 3 to 4 (0-10 scale), between "fairly light" and "somewhat hard" (6-20 scale), or between "moderate" to "somewhat strong" (0-10 scale), is generally appropriate for weight reduction programs, corresponding to 60 to 70 percent of the maximal heart rate, which is equivalent to 45 to 57 percent $\dot{V}O_2$max.[24] During this relative intensity, blood lactate levels generally remain low, allowing the individual to exercise for sustained periods, and free fatty acids are used preferentially as a fuel source.[16,19]

In contrast, exercise rated 13 to 16 (6-20 scale), between "somewhat hard" and "hard," or 4 to 6 (0-10 scale), between "somewhat strong and very strong," is generally considered more appropriate for cardiorespiratory conditioning, corresponding to 70 to 85 percent of maximal heart rate, which is equivalent to 57 to 78 percent $\dot{V}O_2$max (Figure 3-3).[18] This rela-

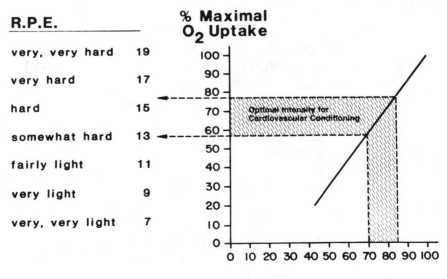

Figure 3-3. Relationships among percentage of maximal oxygen uptake, percentage of maximal heart rate, and Borg's rating of perceived exertion (R.P.E.; 6-20 scale), at the optimal exercise intensity for cardiorespiratory conditioning. (Adapted from Hellerstein, H.K. and B.A. Franklin.)[18]

tive intensity is associated with decreased fat and increased carbohydrate utilization (Figure 3-4).[3] It should be emphasized, however, that the training intensity threshold appears to have a wide variance, and considerable evidence suggests that it increases in direct proportion to the initial level of fitness. Thus, markedly deconditioned adults may show favorable cardiorespiratory adaptation and improvement at initial training intensities that are below theoretically desired target levels.

An American College of Sports Medicine position paper suggests that exercise training programs to improve cardiorespiratory fitness and/or reduce body weight and fat stores include sustained exercise of an endurance nature for at least 20 to 30 minutes duration, an exercise intensity sufficient to expend 300 or more kcal per session, and a minimum of 3 exercise sessions per week.[1] Exercise programs lasting less than 3 months, or those performed twice a week — regardless of the intensity,

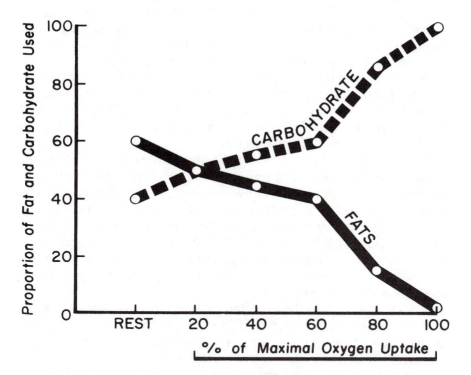

Figure 3-4. Relative contributions from fat and carbohydrate as a function of exercise intensity, expressed as a percentage of the maximal oxygen uptake ($\dot{V}O_2$max). During mild intensity exercise (e.g., below 57 percent $\dot{V}O_2$max), fat serves as an important energy substrate. However, at higher intensities, there is decreased fat and increased carbohydrate utilization. (Adapted from Åstrand, P.O. and K. Rodahl).[3]

duration, or both — are generally ineffective in weight reduction programs.[7,22]

The most effective exercises for the endurance phase employ large muscle groups, are maintained continuously, and are rhythmical and aerobic in nature. Examples include: walking, jogging (in place or moving), running, stationary or outdoor cycling, swimming, skipping rope, rowing, climbing stairs, and stepping on and off a bench. Other exercise modalities commonly used in conditioning programs for the sedentary adult include: calisthenics, particularly those involving sustained total body movement; recreational games; and weight training. The latter is a particularly important option, since traditional aerobic conditioning regimens often fail to accommodate participants who have an interest in improving strength and muscle tone.

Walking has several advantages over other forms of exercise during the initial phase of a physical conditioning program. Brisk walk training programs can result in a substantial increase in aerobic capacity and a reduction in body weight and fat stores, particularly when the walking duration exceeds 30 minutes.[17,23] Walking offers an easily tolerable exercise intensity and causes fewer musculoskeletal and orthopedic problems of the legs, knees, and feet than jogging or running.[23] Moreover, it is a "companionable" activity that requires no special equipment other than a pair of well-fitted athletic shoes. Walking in water[11] or with a backpack[25] offer additional options for those who wish to lose weight and improve fitness.

The gross caloric cost of walking approximates 1.15 kcal/kg/mile (Note: 1 kg = 2.2 pounds) (Figure 3-5).[15] Furthermore, unless the individual walks at extremely slow or fast paces (i.e., less than 1.9 mph or more than 3.7 mph), the caloric cost per mile is relatively independent of speed, increasing linearly as a function of body weight (Figure 3-6).[2] Although many sedentary adults may be unable to maintain a jog or run, they can expend substantial amounts of energy by moving their body weights over considerable distances.

As a variation to the standard walking format, several other activities can also be used during the endurance phase. For example, instead of 30 to 40 minutes of walking alone, a 15-minute walk may be supplemented by 15 to 25 minutes of simple relays, contests, and individual, group, or partner activities. During the simple relays and contests, participants are grouped homogeneously. Individuals with comparable aerobic fitness are teamed with others who have similar performance abilities. A variety of stations or circuit type work are examples of methods that lend themselves to the individual control of energy expendi-

Kcal/Kg/Mile

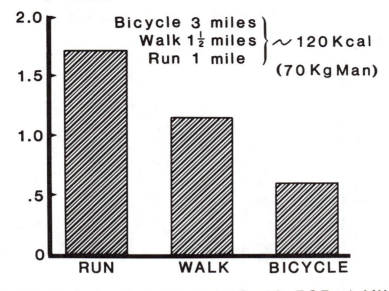

GROSS ENERGY REQUIREMENTS FOR 1 MILE

Figure 3-5. Comparison of the gross energy requirements for running, walking, and outdoor bicycling. The energy cost per mile for walking falls between that of running and bicycling: 1.15 kcal/kg/mile. Expressed another way, the energy cost of walking 1.5 miles is equivalent to bicycling 3 miles or running 1 mile. (Adapted from Franklin, B.A. and M. Rubenfire.)[15]

ture. The exercise leader may frequently change the style of a relay to include handling of sport balls, foot dribbling, or a combination of foot dribbling and hand maneuvers. As a variation, members of the class may work in groups of 2, 3, 4, and perhaps as many as 8.

During the endurance phase of the program, the exercise leader relies heavily upon the regulation of exercise intensity via heart rate and perceived exertion monitoring.[8] Each participant must internalize the feeling of his/her energy expenditure. Frequent heart rate counts of 10-seconds duration (multiplied by 6) or 15-seconds duration (multiplied by 4) act as checks as well as reinforcements to the participant that he/she is exercising within a safe and effective intensity range.

Heart rate is most commonly monitored via palpation of the radial (wrist) artery. Excessive pressure when monitoring heart rate via the carotid (neck) artery can produce bradycardia (slowing of the heart rate),[18] yielding an inaccurate estimate of the relative exercise intensity. This is eliminated when adult exercisers are taught how to palpate the carotid artery correctly.[20]

The exercise leader may choose to lead participants in a

GROSS CALORIC REQUIREMENTS
PER MILE FOR WALKING

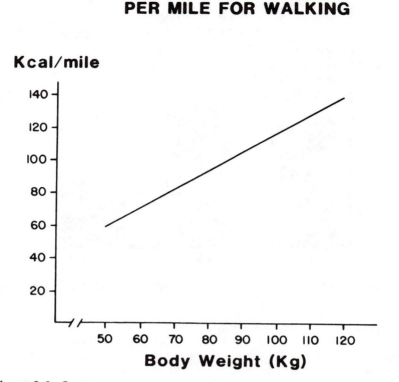

Figure 3-6. Gross caloric requirements per mile of walking, expressed as a function of body weight. Unless the individual walks at extremely slow or fast paces (i.e., less than 1.9 mph or greater than 3.7 mph), the caloric cost per mile is relatively independent of speed, increasing linearly as a function of body weight.

variety of individual activities during the endurance phase. Many forms of human locomotion may be employed, including: walking, striding, jogging, skipping (forward, rearward, sideward), crawling (if mats are available), and hopping (short period of time). In addition to the locomotor task, participants may carry sport balls, foot or hand dribble them, air dribble them, or bounce them off supporting walls. In addition to endurance, gross motor skills are developed. These skills are used in the games portion, which follows the endurance phase of the program.

Rationale for Arm Exercise Training

Numerous studies have investigated the physiological adaptations of trained versus untrained muscles to regular endurance exercise. Results have generally shown that the favorable cardiovascular, respiratory, and metabolic adaptations to exercise training are largely *specific* to the muscle groups that have been trained. For example, a classic Scandinavian study demonstrated that leg training caused a substantial decrease in the heart rate response to leg exercise, but not to arm exercise. Conversely, arm training resulted in a marked reduction in the heart rate response to arm exercise, but not to leg exercise.[9] Similar "muscle specific" adaptations have been shown for other physiologic variables. These findings imply that a substantial portion of the conditioning response is attributed to adaptations in the trained muscles alone.

The limited degree of crossover of training benefits from one set of limbs to another appears to discredit the general practice of restricting exercise training to the legs alone (e.g., walking, jogging, stationary cycle ergometry).[13] Many recreational and occupational activities require arm work to a greater extent than leg work. Consequently, exercisers who rely on their upper extremities should be advised to train the arms as well as the legs, with the expectation of an improved capacity for both forms of effort.

Specially designed arm ergometers are particularly good for upper extremity training. Other equipment suitable for upper body training includes rowing machines, weight training apparatus, wall pulleys, combined arm/leg ergometers, and simulated cross-country skiing devices. Various sport and recreational activities can also be utilized for upper extremity training, including canoeing, swimming, and cross-country skiing. Specific precautions should be taken during the latter, particularly with cardiac patients, as physiological responses such as heart rate are frequently inordinately high and do not correspond with ratings of perceived exertion.[21]

GAMES

During the games portion of the program (5 to 10 minutes), a wide variety of improvised or mutually satisfying activities are presented (see Chapter 11 for ideas and details). *The purpose of this program option is to provide participants with recreational opportunities and to permit them to express themselves physically.* Modified forms of volleyball similar to Newcomb or bounce ball are played, with little concern about standards of perfection that permeate activities with specific rules and regulations. For example, if nets are used as barriers, they may be at lower heights than standard official tournament or regulation play. Likewise, overt infractions to play are secondary to play itself. Often participants move freely from side to side or team to team in an effort to encourage "play," rather than to score points or secure a team victory. Many games may be of a nonsense variety but require a moderate degree of physical dexterity. Physical skills are developed and nurtured during the games portion of the fitness program.

The exercise leader has a responsibility to positively reinforce individual and team play. At no time should individuals, teams, or sides be reprimanded for what would be considered violations of competitive play in regulation games. The emphasis of the games portion is enjoyment rather than a high level of individual or team competition.[27] Heart rates should still be monitored periodically.

COOL-DOWN

The cool-down (5 minutes) provides a gradual recovery from the intensity of the stress of the 2 previous phases — endurance and games. Exercises of a muscle-stretching or muscle-lengthening nature are encouraged. Special attention should be paid to the extensor muscles of the back, lower legs, and upper extremities. Such "low-level" activities permit appropriate circulatory readjustments and return of the heart rate and blood pressure to near resting values; enhance venous return, thereby reducing the potential for postexercise lightheadedness; facilitate the dissipation of body heat; promote more rapid removal of lactic acid than stationary recovery;[6] and combat the potential deleterious effects of the postexercise rise in plasma catecholamines.[10]

During exercise, vasodilation in the active muscles accommodates the blood flow necessary for increased metabolic demands. The potential for accumulation of blood in the lower extremities is countered by a "milking action" of the muscles on the veins. This muscle contraction is facilitated by continued slow walking or low-intensity exercise. To further assist in this process, the veins have one-way valves that permit blood flow in an upward direction only (Figure 3-7). With abrupt cessation of exercise, there is no muscle pump action to return blood to the heart. Consequently, blood may pool in the legs. The subsequent decrease in venous return to the brain, heart, or intestines may result in dizziness or fainting, heart rhythm irregularities, or nausea.[28] *It is critical that the exercise leader insures that partic-*

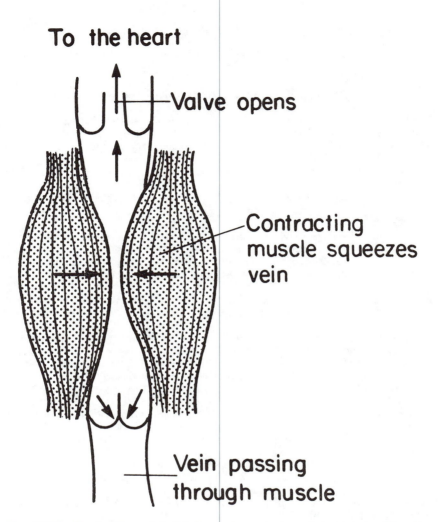

To the heart

Valve opens

Contracting muscle squeezes vein

Vein passing through muscle

Figure 3-7. Contraction of skeletal muscle squeezes veins, pumping blood toward the heart. One-way valves prevent the blood from flowing backward.

ipants continue to move during the cool-down period. The leader should also observe the participants during the recovery phase of the program and encourage adequate circulatory system adjustments prior to their departures.

BIBLIOGRAPHY

1. American College of Sports Medicine. (1978) "Position Statement on the Recommended Quantity and Quality of Exercise for Developing and Maintaining Fitness in Healthy Adults." *Med. Sci. Sports*, 10:7-11.
2. American College of Sports Medicine. (1986) *Guidelines for Graded Exercise Testing and Exercise Prescription*. 3rd ed., Philadelphia: Lea and Febiger.

3. Åstrand, P.O. and K. Rodahl. (1970) *Textbook of Work Physiology*. New York: McGraw-Hill Book Company.

4. Barnard, R.J., G.W. Gardner, N.V. Diaco, et al. (1973) "Cardiovascular Responses to Sudden Strenuous Exercise: Heart Rate, Blood Pressure, and ECG." *J. Appl. Physiol.*, 34:833-837.

5. Barnard, R.J., R. MacAlpin, A.A. Kattus, et al. (1973) "Ischemic Response to Sudden Strenuous Exercise in Healthy Men." *Circulation*, 48:936-942.

6. Belcastro, A.N. and A. Bonen. (1975) "Lactic Acid Removal Rates During Controlled and Uncontrolled Recovery Exercise." *J. Appl. Physiol.*, 39:932-936.

7. Bjorntorp, P. (1978) "Physical Training in the Treatment of Obesity." *Int. J. Obesity*, 2:149-156.

8. Borg, G. (1982) "Psychophysical Bases of Perceived Exertion." *Med. Sci. Sports Exercise*, 14:377-381.

9. Clausen, J.P., J. Trap-Jensen, and N.A. Lassen. (1970) "The Effects of Training on the Heart Rate During Arm and Leg Exercise." *Scand. J. Clin. Lab. Invest.*, 26:295-301.

10. Dimsdale, J.E., H. Hartley, T. Guiney, et al. (1984) "Postexercise Peril: Plasma Catecholamines and Exercise." *J.A.M.A.*, 251:630-632.

11. Evans, B.W., K.J. Cureton and J.W. Purvis. (1978) "Metabolic and Circulatory Responses to Walking and Jogging in Water." *Research Quarterly for Exercise and Sport*, 49:442-449.

12. Foster, C., D.S. Dymond, J. Carpenter, et al. (1982) "Effect of Warm-Up on Left Ventricular Response to Sudden Strenuous Exercise." *J. Appl. Physiol.: Respirat. Environ. Exercise Physiol.*, 53:380-383.

13. Franklin, B.A. (1989) "Aerobic Exercise Training Programs for the Upper Body." *Med. Sci. Sports Exerc.*, 21:S141-148.

14. Franklin, B.A., H.K. Hellerstein, S. Gordon, et al. (1986) "Exercise Prescription for the Myocardial Infarction Patient." *J. Cardiopulmonary Rehabil.*, 6:62-79.

15. Franklin, B.A. and M. Rubenfire. (1980) "Losing Weight Through Exercise. *J.A.M.A.*, 244:377-379.

16. Girandola, R.N. (1976) "Body Composition Changes in Women: Effects of High and Low Exercise Intensity." *Arch. Phys. Med. Rehabil.*, 57:297-300.

17. Gwinup, G. (1975) "Effect of Exercise Alone on the Weight of Obese Women." *Arch. Intern. Med.*, 135:676-680.

18. Hellerstein, H.K. and B.A. Franklin. (1984) "Exercise Testing and Prescription." In Wenger, N.K. and H.K. Hellerstein (eds.): *Rehabilitation of the Coronary Patient*. 2nd ed., New York, John Wiley, pp. 197-284.

19. Katch, F.I. and W.D. McArdle. (1977) *Nutrition, Weight Control, and Exercise*. Boston: Houghton Mifflin.

20. Oldridge, N.B., W.L. Haskell, and P. Single. (1981) "Carotid Palpation, Coronary Heart Disease and Exercise Rehabilitation." *Med. Sci. Sports Exerc.*, 13:6-8.

21. Oldridge, N.B., and C. Connolly. (1989) "Oxygen Uptake and Heart Rate During Cross-Country Skiing and Track Walking after Myocardial Infarction." *Am. Heart J.*, 117:495-497.

22. Pollock, M.L., J. Wilmore and S.M. Fox. (1978) *Health and Fitness Through Physical Activity*. New York: John Wiley.

23. Pollock, M.L., H.S. Miller, R. Janeway, et al. (1971) "Effects of Walking on Body Composition and Cardiovascular Function of Middle-Aged Men. *J. Appl. Physiol.*, 30:126-130.

24. Sharkey, B.J. (1975) *Physiological Fitness and Weight Control*. Missoula: Mountain Press.

25. Shoenfeld, Y., G. Keren, T. Shimoni, et al. (1980) "Walking: A Method for Rapid Improvement of Physical Fitness." *J.A.M.A.*, 243:2062-2063.

26. Stoedefalke, K.G., and J.L. Hodgson. (1975) "Exercise Rx — Designing a Program." *Medical Opinion*, 4:48-55.

27. Stoedefalke, K.G. (1974) "Physical Fitness Programs for Adults." *Am. J. Cardiol.*, 33:787-790.

28. Zohman, L.R. (1974) Beyond Diet. . . . *Exercise Your Way to Fitness and Heart Health*. Englewood Cliffs, NJ: CPC International Inc.

4

Educational/Motivational Strategies

Exercise compliance appears to be predicated in part on the attainment of two major program objectives: a) educating participants *why* and *how* they should be physically active, and b) motivating them to follow through with a personal physical fitness program.[40] Unfortunately, exercise testing and exercise prescription are often emphasized more than education and motivation. Consequently, negative variables often outweigh the positive variables contributing to sustained participant interest and enthusiasm (Figure 4-1).[8] Such imbalance leads to a decline in adherence as program effectiveness diminishes.

Adult fitness and cardiac exercise programs need to include education as well as selected motivational strategies.[31] These components are responsibilities of the exercise leader.

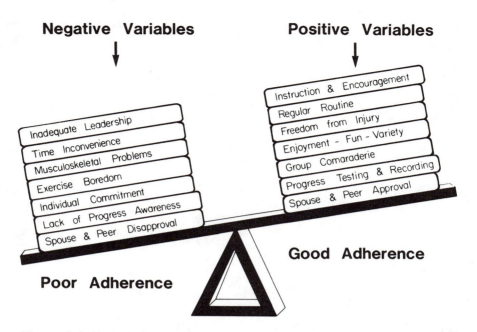

Negative Variables

Positive Variables

Inadequate Leadership
Time Inconvenience
Musculoskeletal Problems
Exercise Boredom
Individual Commitment
Lack of Progress Awareness
Spouse & Peer Disapproval

Instruction & Encouragement
Regular Routine
Freedom from Injury
Enjoyment - Fun - Variety
Group Comaraderie
Progress Testing & Recording
Spouse & Peer Approval

Good Adherence

Poor Adherence

Figure 4-1. Variables affecting compliance to physical conditioning programs. Oftentimes, negative variables outweigh the positive variables, resulting in poor adherence.

EDUCATION

Research suggests that the individual who thoroughly understands the reasons for following a particular lifestyle modification will be more inclined to do so. This was attested to by the overwhelming response to the book *Aerobics*,[4] Kenneth Cooper's effort to inform an educated audience specifically "why" regular exercise is essential to improving general health and well-being. Similarly, the success of the late Jim Fixx's best seller, *The Complete Book of Running*,[7] was attributed in part to the wealth of information that it provided regarding "how" to exercise.

Previously sedentary adults embarking on a physical conditioning program often have unrealistic impressions of safe and effective training practices. The threshold exercise dosage (frequency, intensity, duration) needed to improve fitness is frequently overestimated.[31] Instructors should emphasize that "it does not require pain to make gain." The mode of exercise training must coincide with the exerciser's needs and expectations and be specific in order to enhance the desired fitness component. Otherwise, undue fatigue, extreme muscle soreness, and injury may result with an associated high probability of dropout.

Education stressing both *whys* and *hows* should serve as an integral part of the exercise program and provide substantive information on body mechanics, energy expenditure, cardiovascular health, exercise prescription, the importance of warm-up and cool-down,[35] the concept of perceived exertion,[3] and common exercise myths and misconceptions.[9] Moreover, instruction should include information on appropriate exercise clothing and shoes, nutrition, relaxation techniques, and the effects of ambient temperature and humidity on performance. Finally, participants should be cautioned against certain practices that counteract the benefits of exercise and/or may be potentially hazardous, such as exercise during illness, cold or very hot showers, cigarette smoking, alcohol consumption, ingestion of large meals immediately before or soon after exercise, and spasmodic high intensity exercise bouts.[13]

The educational information that is presented to participants should meet three specific criteria: *catch their attention; be simple; and, be easy to remember and act upon.*[31] Several programmatic options such as films, booklets, and lectures, can be used to promote this program component. Such aids can help give participants a better understanding of the health benefits of regular physical activity. Eye-catching posters, bulletin boards, and educational murals facilitate the dissemination of current literature and human interest stories related to exercise and physical fitness. Such decor motivates exercise behavior and creates an environment that fosters positive feelings. A regular newsletter can also provide information on physical activity, heart disease, weight control, stress, and nutrition. In addition, it serves as a great way to acknowledge participant accomplishments, since most people enjoy seeing their name in print. Finally, periodic meetings with participants and spouses allow for the discussion of topics such as exercise prescription, diet, and weight control. In this format, however, the exercise leader should emphasize those benefits that will have particular significance to individual participants, explaining what it will take to achieve these objectives in terms of both time and effort.

MOTIVATION

In addition to educating people about exercise, it is necessary to motivate them to act. *Motivation is a crucial factor in program effectiveness, safety, and long-term compliance.* Since the magnitude of the conditioning response varies directly with the frequency of participation, poorly motivated subjects (infrequent attenders) are often training failures. Conversely, overly motivated or competitive subjects often overestimate their capacities and are thus subject to orthopedic complications, muscle soreness, or both. Thus, poorly or overly motivated subjects may become exercise program dropouts.[20]

To understand why people sometimes lack the motivation for regular physical activity, one must first acknowledge a simple, yet important fact: exercise is voluntary and time-consuming. Accordingly, exercise may extend the day or compete with other valued interests and responsibilities of daily life.[31] While most persons can be moved to start an exercise program, motivating the individual to continue is often a difficult task. To maintain an exercise commitment the individual must develop a positive attitude toward exercise that reinforces adherence. *This is particularly important over the initial 90 days of participation during which time dropout is most likely to occur.*[36] Accordingly, activity leaders must allow for differences in attitude toward exercise and prescribe programs that meet individual needs.

Several motivational variables in program design (Figure

MOTIVATION
O PINION AND ATTITUDE

T HERAPEUTIC

I NSTRUCTORS

V ARIATION

A EROBIC

T EAM APPROACH

I NVOLVEMENT

O BJECTIVE TESTING

N ONCOMPETITIVE

Figure 4-2. Motivational approaches to exercise programming that may lead to improved attendance and a decreased dropout rate.

4-2) may enhance regular attendance and facilitate increased adherence. However, the motivation to continue in an exercise program is specific to that individual. What is meaningful and motivates one participant may be meaningless to another. The exercise leader should realize that if program modifications or motivational techniques affect even a small percentage of the participants, they are worthwhile.[31]

Motivating people to initiate and maintain an exercise commitment is a learned process that involves understanding what triggers human behavior. Research and empirical observation suggest that selected exercise program modifications and motivational strategies may enhance participant interest, enthusiasm, and long-term compliance.[8,10,21,37] These include:

- *Pay attention to the exercise facilities and locker rooms*. One of the first things exercisers notice is the cleanliness of the fitness facilities. Comfortably bright lights, light-colored walls, and bright carpets all suggest a clean environment. Shower and changing areas should be sanitized daily. In addition, the facility should have a good ventilation system and control over temperature and humidity. Regular maintenance for all exercise equipment should be standard procedure.

- *Clarify individual needs to establish the appropriate exercise prescription*. A preliminary semistructured interview allows one to determine exactly what the client expects from the exercise program. During this interview the exercise leader should discuss individual needs and expectations, set reasonable short- and long-term goals, and establish a schedule to monitor and renegotiate progress.[31] Clear-cut steps should be established that gradually move the participant toward a program of regular exercise. The interview also provides a valuable opportunity to learn what individuals enjoy doing in their leisure time. A good strategy is to explain how the fitness program could enhance their recreational performance. For example, perhaps you have a tennis enthusiast. By incorporating into the exercise program a few "personalized" stretching and strengthening exercises for the muscles used in tennis, you create an intrinsic motive to train.

- *Establish short-term goals, rather than emphasizing long-term objectives*. The key is to draw the clients' focus away from final endpoints — a body weight of 170 pounds or a cholesterol level under 200. Participants should be oriented toward intermediate steps that are both realistic and attainable — a principle tenet of sound goal setting. According to Rejewski and Kenney,[31] goal setting needs to be viewed much like climbing a ladder, with an emphasis placed on reasonable distances between rungs. In addition, goals should be specific and clearly defined.

- *Minimize injury with a moderate exercise prescription.* An exercise prescription that is inherently punitive or at odds with a participants' physical or psychological tolerance serves no useful purpose. Inordinate exercise demands, particularly during the initial weeks of a physical conditioning program, often result in muscle soreness, orthopedic injury, and attrition. The exercise leader should recognize that excessive frequency (more than 5 days/week) and duration (more than 45 minutes/session) of training offer the participant little additional gain in aerobic capacity ($\dot{V}O_2max$), whereas the incidence of orthopedic injury increases disproportionately (Figure 4-3).[30] Similarly, high-intensity training (exceeding 90 percent

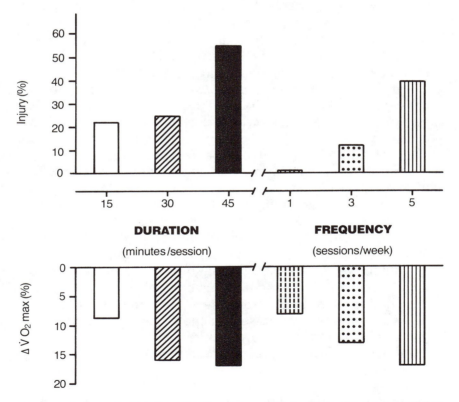

Figure 4-3. Relationship between frequency and duration of exercise training, improvement in aerobic capacity ($\dot{V}O_2max$), and the incidence of orthopedic injury. Above an exercise duration of 30 minutes/session, or a frequency of 3 sessions/week, additional improvement in $\dot{V}O_2max$ is small, yet the injury rate increases disproportionately. (Adapted from Pollock, M.L., et al.)[30]

VO_2max) provides little additional improvement in cardio-respiratory function, and is associated with an injury rate of at least 50 percent.[14,15] A recommended program for beginners is to exercise 20 to 30 minutes every other day, at an intensity of 40 to 70 percent VO_2max, at a perceived exertion of "fairly light." During this initial adjustment phase there should be little or no emphasis on productivity. Attention to warm-up, proper foot wear, and running terrain (avoiding hard and uneven running surfaces) should also aid in decreasing attrition due to injury.

- *Encourage group participation*. Poorer long-term exercise compliance has been reported in programs where one exercises alone as compared to those which incorporate group dynamics.[19,39] Nine out of every 10 people prefer group as opposed to individual exercise.[12] Social reinforcement through camaraderie and companionship are potent motivators related to increased exercise compliance.

- *Avoid overemphasis of regimented calisthenics*. Calisthenics, when relied upon too heavily in an exercise program, readily become monotonous and boring, leading to poor exercise adherence. This fact was demonstrated by the 70 percent dropout rate encountered by the Federal Aviation Agency in an exercise study involving 1,244 employees.[6] Similarly, persons who initiate regimented calisthenic programs, frequently become bored and fail to persist with their exercises.

    If "variety is the spice of life," the realm of exercise programming is no exception. The most successful programs offer many options in the conditioning format. Programs should include at least one major activity that each participant enjoys.

    The "Games-As-Aerobics" approach (see Chapter 5) provides an ideal complement to a walk-jog format. The approach differs from many standard intervention or rehabilitation programs in that it maximizes the pleasure principle.[38]

- *Incorporate effective behavioral and programmatic techniques into the physical conditioning program*. Flexibility in goal setting provides the greatest potential for long-term success. Exercise adherence is enhanced through a comprehensive preliminary orientation (i.e., what can be expected) and personalized positive feedback to participants, as well as through longer time-based distance goals, established by the exerciser.[16,17,22] Research has also demonstrated the effectiveness of self-management strategies, including behavioral contracting and goal setting, in improving exercise adherence.[5,23,24] One clear advantage of these techniques is that the participant plays a major role in the planning. Because of the prevalence of coronary heart disease as a principal cause of morbidity and mortality, and the now common use of exercise as a method of primary and secondary prevention, such strategies may have a profound impact on cardiovascular and public health outcomes.[24,25]

- *Employ periodic testing to assess the participant's response to the training program.* Periodic testing with immediate feedback of positive results provides an excellent way to motivate adults to continue participation in an exercise program.[8,24] This feedback must be based on objective methods of evaluation that are sensitive to even minor changes in improvement. Exercise testing, body composition assessment, and serum lipid profiling should be performed prior to the physical conditioning program and at 6- to 12-month intervals to assess the individual's response to the exercise stimulus.[35,37] Favorable adaptations that are often powerful motivators toward continued and renewed enthusiasm and dedication include a decreased heart rate and systolic blood pressure at rest and at standard submaximal workloads, decreased percent body fat, reduced cholesterol and triglyceride levels, increased high density lipoprotein (HDL) cholesterol, and improved aerobic capacity. These data and other test results can be transformed into a risk factor profile (Table 4–1) to provide an excellent means of ensuring positive reinforcement. Simple self-administered monitoring of the resting pulse rate should also be encouraged, as progress can often be seen during the initial weeks of a training regimen.

Both submaximal and maximal exercise testing have been employed to assess serial changes in cardiovascular fitness over time. The submaximal test, or mini-test, is particularly easy to administer and requires no physician supervision. The baseline exercise test protocol is followed, allowing a comparison of the heart rate, blood pressure, and rating of perceived exertion[3] at identical submaximal workloads. The endpoint of the test is the workload at which the peak training heart rate has been achieved. Aerobic capacity can be estimated by plotting the mini-test heart rate versus workload relationship; the latter is expressed in metabolic equivalents (METs) (1 MET = 3.5 ml O_2/kg body weight/min) extrapolated to the maximum heart rate attained on initial exercise testing (Figure 4–4). Self-monitored, submaximum mini-tests are effective in improving program adherence by involving participants in the decision-making process with regard to exercise progression.[23,27,28]

Workloads	Mini-Test			Initial Test (Pre-conditioning)		
	Heart Rate	Blood Pressure	RPE	Heart Rate	Blood Pressure	RPE
Rest	64	106/74		59	120/78	
2.0 mph 0% grade	68	122/70	6	94	130/78	11
3.0 mph 0% grade	76	132/74	7	113	158/78	14
3.0 mph 2.5% grade	80	136/80	9	120	170/78	15-16
3.0 mph 5.0% grade	86	142/78	9-10	125	182/78	17
3.0 mph 7.5% grade	98	146/82	12			
3.0 mph 10% grade	106	148/80	13-14			

Estimated Peak Mets After Phase II Exercise Program – From mini test results

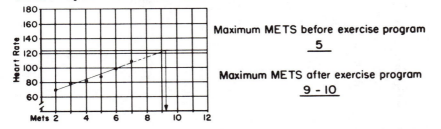

Maximum METS before exercise program

5

Maximum METS after exercise program

9 - 10

Figure 4-4. Comparison of heart rate, blood pressure, and rating of perceived exertion (RPE) to identical submaximal workloads during "mini-testing" versus initial (baseline) exercise testing. Extrapolation of the "mini-test" heart rate/workload (METs) relationship permits estimation of the aerobic capacity, expressed in METs.

- *Organize events for participants, family, and friends.* Lack of social support is frequently found to be a precursor to exercise noncompliance. Accordingly, attention should be focused not only on the participant, but also on family and friends. Spouse support and approval appears to play a key role in this regard. The importance of this influence became evident in one study which investigated the relationship between the wife's attitude toward the exercise program and her husband's adherence in the 18 months' duration of the program. The results showed that the husband's adherence to the exercise program was directly related to the wife's attitude toward it. Eighty percent of those men whose spouses had a positive attitude toward the program demonstrated a good to excellent adherence pattern, contrasted with only 20 percent who exhibited a fair to poor adherence. However, when the spouses' attitudes were neutral or negative, only 40 percent showed good to excellent adherence with the remaining 60 percent having a fair to poor adherence (Figure 4-5).[12] Similar

TABLE 4-1. Risk Factor Profile.

Name _____

Physician _____ Date _____

PERSONAL RISK FACTOR PROFILE

Modifiable Risk Factors	Last Value	Today's Value	Recommended Value	Recommendations
BODY FAT Excessive body fatness is associated with the development of coronary artery disease. Weight loss should be directed towards losing fat not muscle. A combined program of diet and regular exercise is indicated. Weight loss should generally not exceed 2 pounds per week.			Men = 15-18% Women = 22-25%	1. Continue with present program 2. Increase duration and/or frequency of aerobic exercise 3. Lower total caloric intake 4. Reduce body weight
BODY WEIGHT Body weight includes two major components - lean tissue and fat. Your recommended body weight has been calculated to correspond to an "ideal" body fatness: 15-18% for men, or 22-25% for women.				1. Continue with present program 2. Decrease daily caloric intake 3. Increase daily caloric expenditure
CIGARETTE SMOKING* Cigarette smoking is the leading cause of lung cancer and lung-related diseases. It also contributes significantly to high blood pressure, coronary artery disease and strokes.				1. Quit smoking 2. Avoid smoke-filled areas 3. Consider behavior modification classes
REGULAR PHYSICAL EXERCISE Regular aerobic exercise improves the cardiovascular system (heart and lungs). It controls body weight, increases HDL cholesterol, enhances muscle strength and flexibility and may help to prevent osteoporosis (brittle bones).			4 days/week; 45-60 minutes of aerobic exercise	1. Continue with present exercise program
BLOOD PRESSURE* Persons having a consistently elevated blood pressure (resting values above 140/90 mmHg) have an increased risk for atherosclerosis and stroke.			140/90 mmHg or less	1. Continue with present program 2. Consult physician 3. Continue with medications 4. Reduce body weight 5. Lower salt intake 6. Follow exercise prescription 7. Attend stress reduction classes
PSYCHOLOGICAL STRESS High levels of stress and how it is handled *may* be associated with an increased risk for coronary artery disease.				1. Attend stress reduction classes 2. Practice methods of relaxation 3. Regular exercise 4. Practice meditation

* One of the primary risk factors

42   ON THE BALL

TABLE 4-1. (continued)

Name _____

Physician _____ Date _____

PERSONAL RISK FACTOR PROFILE

Modifiable Risk Factors	Last Value	Today's Value	Recommended Value	Recommendations
TOTAL CHOLESTEROL* An elevated blood cholesterol level (above 200 mg/dl) is associated with an increased build up of fatty substances called plaque within the artery wall. This process is referred to as atherosclerosis. The narrowing of these arteries limits the flow of oxygen - carrying blood. If this occurs in the coronary arteries, chest discomfort called angina and/or a heart attack may occur.			200 or less	1. Continue with present program 2. Consult with physician/dietitian 3. Lower intake of whole milk, dairy products, eggs, saturated fats, and red meats 4. Increase fiber and whole grain products
HDL CHOLESTEROL HDL (High Density Lipoprotein) cholesterol is a component of cholesterol. It is often referred to as "good cholesterol", since it helps in the removal of cholesterol from the blood. High levels of HDL (above 40 mg/dl) are associated with a reduced risk for coronary artery disease.			40 or more	1. Continue with present program 2. Follow exercise program regularly 3. Reduce body weight 4. Stop cigarette smoking
CHOLESTEROL/HDL RATIO The ratio of total cholesterol to HDL should be less than 5. This can be calculated by dividing the total cholesterol by the HDL value. If your number is greater than five, you are at increased risk for coronary artery disease.			5.0 or less	1. Continue with present program 2. Decrease total cholesterol level 3. Increase HDL cholesterol level
TRIGLYCERIDES Elevated triglyceride levels (above 140 mg/dl) are linked to obesity, increased sugar or alcohol intake, and an inactive lifestyle. Dietary changes along with regular endurance exercise are helpful in lowering triglyceride levels.			140 or less	1. Continue with present program 2. Consult with physician/dietitian 3. Lower intake of saturated fats, sugar and alcohol 4. Lower total caloric intake 5. Reduce body weight 6. Regular aerobic exercise program
GLUCOSE An elevated blood sugar level (glucose above 110 mg/dl) after a 12 hour fast suggests the potential for diabetes. Diabetes speeds up the rate of atherosclerosis. It is also related to high levels of total cholesterol and triglycerides, increased body weight and low HDL levels.			110 or less	1. See personal physician 2. Follow dietary recommendations prescribed by physician/dietitian 3. Decrease total body weight 4. Regular aerobic exercise program 5. Continue medications

* One of the primary risk factors

POSITIVE

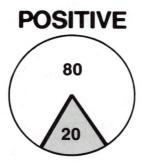

80

20

NEUTRAL OR NEGATIVE

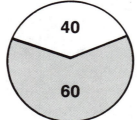

40

60

ADHERENCE PATTERNS

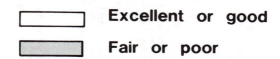

Excellent or good

Fair or poor

Figure 4-5. Relation of wives' attitudes to husbands' adherence to an exercise training program. (Adapted from Heinzelman, F. and R.W. Bagley)[12]

observations have been made in exercise programs designed for cardiac patients.[24,28]

These findings suggest that program counseling and educational gatherings including both participants and spouses will help to create and maintain positive attitudes that support exercise adherence. To this end, cardiac rehabilitation programs should include regularly scheduled social events so that family and friends of patients can meet each other and perhaps share some of the adjustments they have made as a result of the participants' heart disease.

• *Provide progress charts to record exercise achievements.* The importance of immediate positive feedback on health-related behavior is well-documented. A recording system that allows the participant to document daily cumulative exercise achievements (e.g., mileage) can provide a means to this end.[32] For example, the La Crosse Exercise Program "distance drum" provides participants with a record of their accumulated running miles. Even more sophisticated is the computerized exercise session progress report system at the Aerobics Center in Dallas, Texas. The system provides participants with an updated record of the number of "aerobic points" they have earned, the miles they have run, and related exercise accomplishments. The popularity and success of this computer-based system is its basic psychology, a reward system that instantaneously reveals points earned. A practical alternative, however, is a progress chart which allows the exerciser to record his or her daily workout mileage. It tells participants and peers what goals have been accomplished. Furthermore, if the chart is strategically placed near the running track or locker room, it becomes a matter of pride to individuals to "increase" their exercise totals. The result may be fewer missed workouts!

- *Include an optional recreational game to the conditioning program format.* The standard warm-up, endurance phase, cool-down sequence used in most physical conditioning programs offers little in terms of variety or fun. Consequently, a recreational game should be included as an option to this format. Game modifications that serve to minimize skill and competition and maximize participant success are particularly important in adult fitness and cardiac exercise programs. The imaginative exercise leader may suggest a smaller court size, frequent player rotation, intermittent play, subtle rule changes, or adjusted scorekeeping. For example, volleyball played allowing one bounce of the ball per side, facilitates longer rallies and provides additional fun, while minimizing the skill level required to appreciate the game. Many team games and individual sports can be modified in a similar fashion. Through such modifications, the leader is better able to emphasize the primary goal of the activity: enjoyment of the game for its own sake.[35]

- *Establish regularity of workouts.* Starting the exercise session at the same time each day automatically eliminates the battle one has to wage as to when to start the workout. If adults get into the habit of starting workouts at a certain time at regular intervals, they will accept them as part of their routine schedules and not just something to do if "free" time is available. Exercise will become habitual, and certain days won't seem complete without it. The exercise leader should select a certain time or times of the day, preferably early morning and/or early evening, to offer the physical conditioning sessions. Availability of both morning and evening sessions should accommodate the varied schedules of participants.[11]

- *Play music during exercise sessions.* Compliance may be improved by systematically distracting the individuals' attention away from the discomforts that may be produced by exercise. Perhaps the most widely used dissociative technique is music.[31] However, background music should be targeted to the participants (e.g., big band) and not the staff. Music may mask general fatigue, enhance mood, and stimulate participants to exercise more energetically.[33,34] This notion was substantiated in a survey in which 99 out of 114 joggers (87 percent) indicated a preference for background music during their training.[8] Many felt that inspiring music aided their workouts; others perceived reductions in their ratings of exertion at any given pace.

- *Recognize individual accomplishments through a system of extrinsic rewards.* Recognition of achievements, in the form of certificates, inexpensive plastic trophies, plaques, or T-shirts, can be valuable incentives as long as they are not perceived by participants as manipulative. When extrinsic rewards are viewed as positive reinforcement — "you deserve recognition" — they are likely to be well-received. A yearly fitness awards ceremony, including spouses, provides an opportunity to recognize accomplishments related to improved general health and exercise performance. Special award categories may include smoking cessation, best exercise attendance, most improved fitness, greatest weight or body fat loss, and best or most improved volleyball player. Awards for these and related categories can be meaningful and powerful motivators producing renewed interest and enthusiasm.

    It should be emphasized, however, that compliance problems may arise when behavior becomes driven by extrinsic motives, if the rewards are no longer available.[31] Accordingly, extrinsic rewards should be selectively employed or, at the very least, integrated with intrinsic rewards that are inherent to the person's experience.

- *Provide quality, enthusiastic exercise leaders.* Although numerous variables affect participant exercise compliance, perhaps the most important is the exercise leader. Exercise leaders should be well-trained, highly motivated, innovative, and enthusiastic.[21,26,27] Certain leadership traits and skills that appear to be particularly important are listed in Table 4–2. The

TABLE 4-2. Traits and Skills of the Successful Exercise Leader

Traits	Skills
Regard for fellow leaders	Ability to establish rapport
Alert to social environment	Articulate orally and in writing
Cooperative	Creative and innovative
Decisive	Knowledgeable-intelligent
Dependable	Organized
Empathetic	Physically talented
Flexible	Tactful
Energetic-enthusiastic	Adapts programs when appropriate
Self-confident	
Willing to assume responsibility	

exercise leader is a very visible person. He or she must appear fit and well groomed. Some sort of uniform dress is also mandatory.

Specific behavioral objectives of the fitness instructor or exercise specialist are outlined by the American College of Sports Medicine (ACSM).[1] Continuing education workshops and certification programs have been developed by the ACSM and Aerobics and Fitness Association of America to promote "quality control" and knowledge and proficiency standards for personnel involved in the administration and leadership of adult fitness and cardiac exercise programs.

Too often, poor participant motivation is identified as the primary reason for lack of compliance with an exercise program. However, two other variables may also be responsible — namely, *poor exercise leadership, inappropriate exercise programming, or both.*

Exercise leadership requires more than directing physical activity. The participants and their individual needs should receive the highest priority.[18] Physical activity programs can satisfy many individual needs including: mastery, attention, recognition, social acceptance, security of health, and social interaction.

The exercise leader should program activities to correspond to stages of the life cycle.[31] For individuals who are in their 20s or early 30s, physical challenges strengthen the ego and serve as a buffer against stress. Such participants often view exercise as a means of controlling weight and improving appearance. From the mid-30s through the 50s, health and the avoidance of cardiovascular disease become potentially powerful motivators. Finally, clients who are in their 60s and 70s often view exercise as a means of counteracting the inevitable decline in function that accompanies biological aging.

An exercise leader must also be able to incorporate fun or play elements into physical conditioning programs. Alternative activities that change the pace of exercise sessions are helpful. Too often, leaders conduct the same activities in the same way because it is comfortable for them. Boredom and, eventually, dissatisfaction, often result.

Exercise leaders are presented the challenge of providing beneficial and enjoyable physical activity for the individuals they serve. This can be accomplished by increasing the physical skills of the participants and by instilling in them a positive attitude toward exercise and recreation. To this end, the exercise leader must possess a knowledge of a variety of physical activities, recognize individual differences and adapt programs accordingly, motivate participants to make a long-term exercise commitment, and cultivate personal associations. *The relationship between the exercise leader and the participant appears to be particularly important.* Table 4-3 lists recommended behavioral strategies of the good exercise leader. The desired outcome of incorporating these strategies into a program is to enhance compliance; that this occurs has been demonstrated in exercise programs for both healthy subjects and cardiac patients.[10,16,17,25,28,29]

TABLE 4-3. Behavioral Strategies of the Good Exercise Leader

1. Show a sincere interest in the participants. Learn why they have gotten involved in your program, and what they would really like to achieve.

2. Be enthusiastic in your instruction and guidance.

3. Develop a personal association and relationship with each participant; exchange names and be sure to shake hands.

4. Consider the various reasons why adults exercise (i.e., health, recreation, weight loss, social, personal appearance) and allow for individual differences.

5. Initiate participant follow-up (e.g., postcards or telephone calls) when several unexplained absences occur in succession. Novice exercisers should be advised that an inevitable slip in attendance does not imply failure.

6. Practice what you preach. Participate in the exercise sessions yourself. Good posture and grooming are essential to projecting the desired self-image. Cigarette smoking should be prohibited, and drinking soda or eating candy on the gymnasium floor should also be unacceptable.

7. Honor special days (e.g., birthdays) or exercise accomplishments with extrinsic rewards such as t-shirts, ribbons, or certificates.

8. Attend personally to orthopedic and musculoskeletal problems. Provide alternatives to floor exercise.

9. Counsel participants on proper foot apparel and exercise clothing.

10. Avoid constant references to complicated medical or physiological terminology, but don't ignore it altogether. Concentrate on a few selected terms to provide a little education at a time.

11. Arrange for occasional visits by personal physicians.

12. Provide a constant flow of newspaper or magazine articles to the participants on topics related to physical activity, and other pertinent information.

13. Encourage an occasional visitor or participant to lead activity.

14. Have a designated area for participant counseling and pay some attention to decor. Also, avoid trying to converse with clients while performing another task simultaneously.

15. Display your continuing education certifications and educational degrees. You are more likely to be successful at modifying behavior if you are perceived to be an expert.

16. Introduce "first-time" exercisers on the gymnasium floor or in the locker room. This orientation will encourage a sense of belonging to the group.

17. Reinforce participants by complimenting them on their appearance as they are exercising. Your conversation during exercise can also serve as a distractor from any unpleasant sensations that they may be experiencing.

18. Consider entering city- or business-sponsored road races to pace your participants. Exercise leaders can also show their interest and enthusiasm by cheering clients at community fitness events.

BIBLIOGRAPHY

1. American College of Sports Medicine. (1986) *Guidelines for Graded Exercise Testing and Exercise Prescription*. 3rd ed., Philadelphia: Lea and Febiger.
2. Andrew, G.M., N.B. Oldridge, J.O. Parker, et al. (1981) "Reasons for Dropout 'from' Exercise Programs for Post-coronary Patients." *Med. Sci. Sports Exerc.*, 13:164-168.
3. Borg, G. (1982) "Psychophysical Bases of Perceived Exertion." *Med. Sci. Sports Exerc.*, 14:377-381.
4. Cooper, K. (1968) *Aerobics*. New York: Bantam Books.
5. Epstein, L., J. Thompson and R. Wing. (1980) "The Effects of Contract and Lottery Procedures on Attendance and Fitness in Aerobic Exercise." *Behavior Modification*, 4:465-479.
6. "Fitness Programs Held Beneficial." (1965) *Medical Tribune*, March, p. 29.
7. Fixx, J. (1977) *The Complete Book of Running*. New York: Random House.
8. Franklin, B.A. (1978) "Motivating and Educating Adults to Exercise." *J. Phys. Ed. Rec.* 49:13-17.
9. Franklin, B.A. (1984) "Myths and Misconceptions in Exercise for Weight Control." In Storlie, J. and H.A. Jordon (eds.): *Nutrition and Exercise in Obesity Management*. New York: Spectrum Publications, Inc., pp. 53-92.
10. Franklin, B.A. (1988) "Program Factors That Influence Exercise Adherence: Practical Adherence Skills for the Clinical Staff." In Dishman, R. (ed.): *Exercise Adherence: Its Impact on Public Health*. Champaign: Human Kinetics Books, pp. 237-258.
11. Franklin, B., E. Buskirk, J. Hodgson, et al. (1979) "Effects of Physical Conditioning on Cardiorespiratory Function, Body Composition and Serum Lipids in Relatively Normal-Weight and Obese Middle-Aged Women." *Intl. J. Obesity*, 3:97-109.
12. Heinzelman, F. and R.W. Bagley. (1970) "Response to Physical Activity Programs and Their Effects on Health Behavior." *Public Health Rep.*, 85:905-911.
13. Hellerstein H.K., E.Z. Hirsch, R. Ader, et al. (1973) "Principles of Exercise Prescription for Normals and Cardiac Subjects." In Naughton, J.P. and H.K. Hellerstein (eds.): *Exercise Testing and Exercise Training in Coronary Heart Disease*. New York: Academic Press, pp. 129-167.
14. Kilbom, A., L. Hartley, B. Saltin, et al. (1969) "Physical Training in Sedentary Middle-Aged and Older Men. I. Medical Evaluation." *Scand. J. Clin. Lab. Invest.*, 24:315-322.
15. Mann, G., H. Garrett, A. Farhi, et al. (1969) "Exercise to Prevent Coronary Heart Disease: An Experimental Study of the Effects of Training on Risk Factors for Coronary Disease in Man." *Am. J. Med.*, 46:12-27.
16. Martin, J.E. and P.M. Dubbert. (1982) "Exercise Applications and Promotion in Behavioral Medicine. Current Status and Future Directions." *J. Consult. Clin. Psychol.*, 50:1004-1017.
17. Martin, J.E. (1989) "Strategies to Enhance Patient Exercise Compliance." In Franklin, B.A., S. Gordon and G.C. Timmis (eds.): *Exercise in Modern Medicine*. Baltimore: Williams and Wilkins, pp. 280-291.
18. Maslow, A.H. (1943) "A Theory of Human Motivation." *Psychol. Rev.*, 50:370-396.
19. Massie, J.F. and R.J. Shephard. (1971) "Physiological and Psychological Effects of Training — A Comparison of Individual and Gymnasium Programs, With a Characterization of the Exercise 'Drop-Out'." *Med. Sci. Sports*, 3:110-117.
20. McHenry, M.M. (1974) "Medical Screening of Patients With Coronary Artery Disease-Criteria for Entrance into Exercise Conditioning Programs." *Am. J. Cardiol.*, 33:752-756.
21. Oldridge, N.B. and K.G. Stoedefalke. (1984) "Compliance and Motivation in Cardiac Exercise Programs." In Franklin, B.A. and M. Rubenfire (eds.): *Symposium on Cardiac Rehabilitation, Clinics in Sports Medicine*. Philadelphia: W.B. Saunders, pp. 443-454.
22. Oldridge, N.B. and J. Spencer. (1985) "Exercise Habits and Perceptions Before and After Graduating or Dropout from Supervised Cardiac Exercise Rehabilitation." *J. Cardiac Rehabil.*, 5:313-319.
23. Oldridge, N.B. and N. Jones. (1981) "Contracting As A Strategy to Reduce Drop Out in Exercise Rehabilitation." *Med. Sci. Sports*, 13:125-126.

24. Oldridge, N.B. (1982) "Compliance and Exercise in Primary and Secondary Prevention of Coronary Heart Diease: A Review." *Prev. Med.*, 11:56-70.
25. Oldridge, N.B. (1988) "Compliance with Exercise in Cardiac Rehabilitation." In Dishman, R. (ed.): *Exercise Adherence: Its Impact on Public Health*. Champaign, Human Kinetics Books, pp. 283-304.
26. Oldridge, N.B. (1977) "What to Look For in an Exercise Class Leader.' *Phys. Sportsmed.*, 5:85-88.
27. Oldridge, N.B. (1988) "Qualities of an Exercise Leader." In Blair, S.N., P. Painter, R.R. Pate, L.K. Smith, and C.B. Taylor (eds): *American College of Sports Medicine Resource Manual for Guidelines for Graded Exercise Testing and Exercise Prescription*, Philadelphia: Lea and Febiger, pp. 239-243.
28. Oldridge, N.B. and N.L. Jones. (1986) "Preventive Use of Exercise Rehabilitation After Myocardial Infarction." *Acta Med. Scand.*, Suppl 711: 123-129.
29. Oldridge, N.B. (1988) "Cardiac Rehabilitation Programs: Compliance and Compliance-Enhancing Strategies." *Sports Medicine*, 6:42-55.
30. Pollock, M.L., L. Gettman, C. Milesis, et al. (1977) "Effects of Frequency and Duration of Training on Attrition and Incidence of Injury." *Med. Sci. Sports*, 9:31-36.
31. Rejewski, W.J. and E.A. Kenney. (1988) *Fitness Motivation: Preventing Participant Dropout*. Champaign: Life Enhancement Publications.
32. Scherf, J. and B.A. Franklin. (1987) "Exercise Compliance: A Data Documentation System." *JOPERD*, 58(6):26-28.
33. Smith, C.A. and L.W. Morris. (1977) "Differential Effects of Stimulative and Seductive Music on Anxiety, Concentration and Performance." *Psych. Reports*, 41: 1047-1053.
34. Steptoe, A. and S. Cox. (1988) "Acute Effects of Aerobic Exercise on Mood." *Health Psych.*, 7:329-340.
35. Stoedefalke, K.G. (1974) "Physical Fitness Programs for Adults." *Am. J. Cardiol.*, 33:787-790.
36. Stoedefalke, K.G. and J.L. Hodgson. (1975) "Exercise Rx — Designing a Program." *Medical Opinion*, 4:48-55.
37. Stoedefalke, K.G. (1973) "The Principles of Conducting Exercise Programs." In Naughton, J.P. and H.K. Hellerstein (eds.): *Exercise Testing and Exercise Training in Coronary Heart Disease*. New York: Academic Press, pp. 299-305.
38. Stoedefalke, K.G. (1973) "Games as Aerobics: Physical Activity and Games in Programs of Intervention and Rehabilitation." Paper presented at the Chicago Heart Association Conference, Chicago, Illinois.
39. Wilhelmsen, L., H. Sanne, D. Elmfeldt, et al. (1975) "A Controlled Trial of Physical Training After Myocardial Infarction: Effects on Risk Factors, Nonfatal Reinfarction, and Death." *Prev. Med.*, 4:491-508.
40. Wilmore, J.H. (1974) "Individual Exercise Prescription." *Am. J. Cardiol.*, 33:757-759.

5

Fun or Pleasure Principle: The "Games-as-Aerobics" Approach

Regardless of participant motivation, if the exercise program is perceived as unpleasant, boring, or inconvenient, adherence becomes a problem. Since poor exercise compliance is often associated with negative program perceptions, participants should engage in activities that elicit positive ratings on the Feeling Scale — an 11-point scale that ranges from +5 (very good) to –5 (very bad) (Table 5-1).[5] This type of assessment may be helpful in detecting problems like boredom or disssatisfaction with exercise.

TABLE 5-1.

Feeling Scale*
+5 Very good
+4
+3 Good
+2
+1 Slightly good
0 Neutral
−1 Slightly bad
−2
−3 Bad
−4
−5 Very bad

*From Rejewski, W.J. and E.A. Kenney[5]

The "games-as-aerobics approach" provides an ideal complement to an endurance training program. The approach emphasizes fun, pleasure, and repeated success, in contrast to the pain and discomfort associated with traditional adult fitness and cardiac exercise programs. Activities may vary with each workout, being limited only by the creativity of the exercise leader. Stretching and flexibility calisthenics and dynamic aerobic exercises are frequently camouflaged as games, relays, or stunts, incorporating ball passing and other movement skills for variety.[6] The participant exercises at his or her own pace, rather than being directed in a format in which all persons are expected to perform the same activity at the same cadence, as in Marine Corps calisthenics. Complementary equipment may include hula hoops, playground or cage balls (Figure 5-1), jump ropes, parachutes, hand weights, and special arm exercise devices.[3]

The approach differs from conventional exercise programs in that total body movement is greater, maximizing the potential for a negative caloric balance. Participants are required to keep moving for a prescribed period of time. Repeated flexion and extension of the upper and lower limbs and slow walking (i.e., 1.5-2.0 mph) are encouraged even during rest breaks.

GENERAL PRINCIPLES OF CONDUCTING ADULT EXERCISE SESSIONS

A few general principles apply to the use of calisthenics, contests, and relays, including competition, safety, and education.

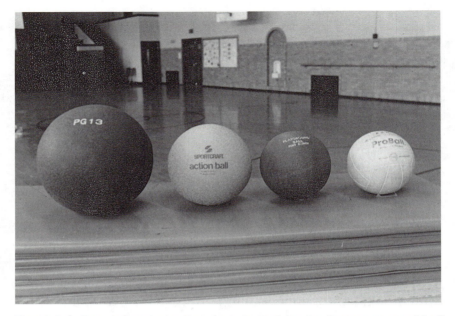

Figure 5-1. Representative exercise equipment for the "games-as-aerobics" approach. A variety of playground balls can be employed in the exercise routines; however, the 8½-inch ball (third from the left) probably has the greatest utility. In addition, large cage balls (2-6 foot diameter) can be used for selected games and relays.

Competition

Time, number of repetitions, and high-intensity activity are not the criteria of a successful exercise session. The challenge to do one's best within the margin of safety is applicable and useful. When individuals, by their very nature, are overly aggressive in their play, they should be addressed after the exercise session or during the workout, if necessary. The need for enjoyable play and participation should exceed artificial standards of perfection in the conduct of the relays and contests.

Safety

In addition to observing participants during the activity session, the exercise leader must concentrate on being safety conscious. Many intervention and rehabilitation program dropouts occur as a result of orthopedic injuries. Some of these orthopedic problems can be avoided simply by reducing the frequency, intensity, and/or duration of training. Potential hazards such as windows, sharp corners, miscellaneous equipment on the gymnasium floor, overenthusiasm, and turning in the wrong direction, are variables that need to be controlled by the program staff. The exercise leader should continually observe participants for signs of fatigue, which invite injury.

Education

The concept of education and instruction should permeate the entire exercise session. Psychologists have shown that people will engage in behaviors that they understand the significance of and believe they can realistically perform.[5] Consequently, exercise leaders should *modify* difficult or strenuous movements, particularly for persons who are starting exercise programs, to insure that the activities are simple enough to perform easily.

Teaching a wide variety of postures and movements requires patience, cooperation, and reinforcement. A previously sedentary middle-aged adult often feels uncomfortable and insecure in performing certain activities. For example, instruction in the use of the foot (medial portion, toe, lateral portion, and heel) and nondominant hand is important. Furthermore, the need for practice should be emphasized. The warming-up and cooling-down phases of the exercise program lend themselves to the acquisition of skills that make the activity program more enjoyable and satisfying. The exercise leader must build on the baseline skill performance of the participant and gradually introduce new activities. The goal is to teach participants to adapt to the intensity of the program while they enjoy success in a variety of basic motor and large muscle activities.

Finally, participants should be discouraged from comparing themselves to or competing with other individuals. Differences in age, habitual physical activity, aerobic capacity, strength and flexibility, and type and extent of disease, invalidate such comparisons and competition. Instead, adult exercisers should realize that each participant has varied objectives that often require different approaches to prescription. If these approaches are followed, the desired effects (if realistic) will occur.

SPECIFIC RECOMMENDATIONS FOR CONDUCTING ADULT EXERCISE SESSIONS[1,2,4]

- Each exercise session must be enjoyable. Fun is an essential ingredient.

- When speaking to a group, be in a position where they can all see and hear you.
- Speak slowly and loudly; enunciate.
- Explain rules clearly.
- Use visual aids when possible and appropriate.
- Give the direction for the movement pattern, i.e., run to the right or clockwise.
- Massive or gross motor activities should dominate the activity session.
- Competition should not be stressed. A favorite side or team should not be permitted to dominate, especially in team games.
- Use the warm-up and cool-down periods to make fitness enjoyable.
- The games portion should be selected on the basis of the physical performance level of the participants. In other words, a low level of organization and activity should dominate. Games should be uncomplicated and have a limited number of rules and few or no penalties for violations. Adjust the rules to fit the size of the group, the playing area, individual performance capability, or equipment available.
- Use well-defined boundary lines.
- Avoid repeated use of elimination-type games.
- Select favorite activities as a treat — use sparingly a favorite game or relay.
- Avoid overlapping areas (when 2 activities are being run simultaneously). Do not present a game-relay that could invite injury as a result of a participant running into a parallel ongoing activity.
- The entire class must be active at the same time. There should be no standing, waiting for turns or unnecessary rest periods. Emphasis must be placed on movement.
- There should be equal turns for all participants in all activities.
- Stop activity at the height of enthusiasm. Adults tend to return to games and movements that they enjoy. Don't succumb to requests for "just one more time" or "let's do it again."
- Be safety conscious — check equipment daily.
- Watch for signs of fatigue and physiological stress. Whenever possible, be in a position to observe the entire exercise area.
- Alternate strenuous with less strenuous games/relays.
- Be creative — imaginative — flexible.
- Show interest and enthusiasm.
- Compliment participants for their behavior in play.
- Evaluate the success of the exercise session, eliminate activities that are not well-received.

BIBLIOGRAPHY

1. Anderson, J. (1968) *Fun With Games*. Madison: Dembar.
2. Anderson, M., E. Elliot, and J. LaBerge. (1966) *Play With a Purpose*. New York: Harper and Row.
3. Frost, G. (1977) "The Playbuoy Exerciser." *Amer. Corr. Therapy J.*, 31:156.
4. Mosston, M. (1965) *Developmental Movement*. Columbus: Merrill.
5. Rejewski, W.J. and E.A. Kenney. (1988) *Fitness Motivation: Preventing Participant Dropout*. Champaign: Life Enhancement Publications.
6. Stoedefalke, K.G. (1973) "Games as Aerobics: Physical Activity and Games in Programs of Intervention and Rehabilitation. " Paper presented at the Chicago Heart Association Conference, Chicago, Illinois.

6

Individual Stationary Activities

The following individual exercises, using a playground ball or volleyball, are primarily designed for the stretching portion of the warm-up and cool-down. For all exercises: Purpose = primary reason for activity and/or focus on muscle groups that are employed; SP = starting position; ES = exercise sequence; and, Note = special considerations and/or modifications.

The number of repetitions of each activity or time allotted for them is left to the exercise leader's discretion. The axiom to remember is, "avoid boredom." The leader should frequently change postures, activities, and expectations, making the exercise sessions dynamic.

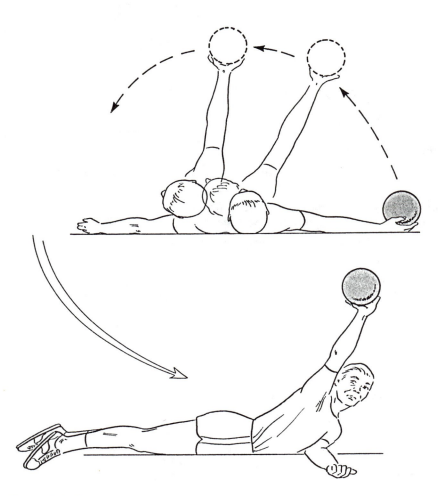

Figure 6-1. Barrel roll.

Purpose: To enhance balance and to improve coordination.

SP: Supine lying position (facing the ceiling) with arm extended and hand holding a ball.

ES: With arm at full extension, roll clockwise or counterclockwise in a complete 360-degree rotation. Change extended arms and repeat the activity.

don't hold breath - BREATHE!

doesn't do what it says

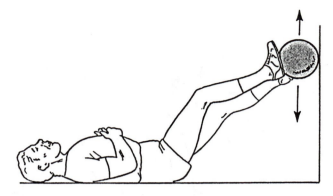

Figure 6-2. Wall walk.

Purpose: To improve abdominal muscle tone and encourage hip flexor activity.

SP: Supine position 2 to 3 feet from a wall. Ball is in contact with the wall and sole of participant's shoes.

ES: Using the sole of the shoe, the ball is moved up and down or left and right.

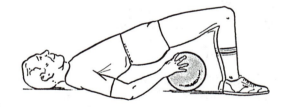

Figure 6-3. Ball circle body.

Purpose: To stretch and tone muscles of the abdomen.

SP: Lie flat on ground with legs flexed at the knee joint and ball at one side of body.

ES: Raise buttocks as shown, push ball to other side of body and lower buttocks. Repeat. Alternatively the ball may be circled around the upper legs without letting the ball touch the ground.

Note: This exercise can be modified into a relay activity using an equal number of participants per side.

do slower
bigger ball
breathe!

stretch but no tone

Stretch is not beyond normal range of motion

doesn't isolate abdominals

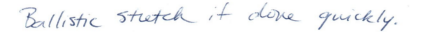

Ballistic stretch if done quickly.

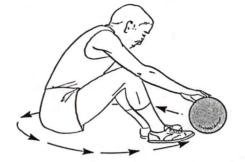

OK

(A)

(B)

Modification:
go over ankles if
flexibility is lacking

Figure 6-4. Trunk flexion with legs flexed at the knee joint (A), or extended (B).

OK Purpose: To stretch the posterior thigh and back muscles, and to improve the mobility of the arm-shoulder joint.

SP: Sitting position with the legs flexed at the knee joint (A) or extended (B). The ball is located at the side of the participant to initiate the movement.

ES: With finger tip control move the ball clockwise or counterclockwise in a 360-degree circle. Controlling hand is changed at the mid-line forward or rearward.

Sugges-
tion: Additional trunk lateral rotation will occur when both hands are placed on the ball using finger tip control.

- More rotation Better.

INDIVIDUAL STATIONARY ACTIVITIES 61

Good for all populations except
low back problems

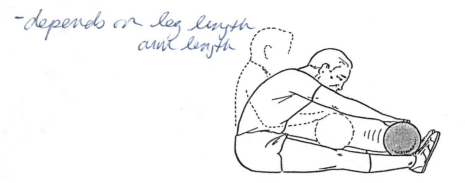

depends on leg length and arm length

Figure 6-5. Trunk flexion with ball.

Purpose: To stretch the posterior thigh muscles and improve trunk flexion.

SP: Sitting position with legs extended and a ball placed on the anterior thighs.

ES: With finger tip control move the ball the length axis of the legs (i.e., toward the toes) by rounding the upper back and flexing the trunk. Return to the starting position and repeat the movement.

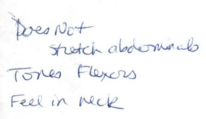

Does Not stretch abdominals
Tones Flexors
Feel in Neck

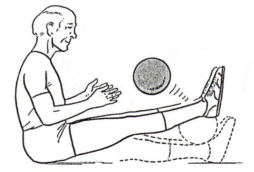

Figure 6-6. Seated leg flick.

Purpose: To stretch and tone muscles of the abdomen.

SP: Seated, legs extended, feet together, ball balanced in the anterior portion of lower legs and feet.

ES: Lift the extended legs with a rapid movement, flicking the ball into your hands.

Note: Starting position can be lying on back rather than seated.

Better But Worse For Back

Note: This activity can be carried out with a partner when sitting side by side. Rather than flicking the ball vertically upward, it can be flicked to the partner's hands.

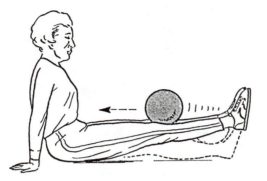

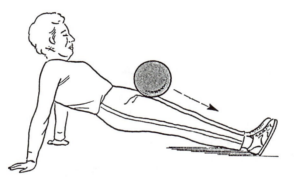

Figure 6-7. Seated ball-leg-roll.

No Ab Stretch
Abs only as stabilizes

Purpose: To stretch and tone muscles of the abdomen.

SP: Seated, legs extended, feet together, ball balanced in anterior portion of lower legs and feet.

ES: Lift extended legs up and allow ball to roll to abdomen. Pick ball up and reach forward to replace on lower legs.

or

Alternatively lift buttocks off ground, allowing ball to roll back down to starting position.

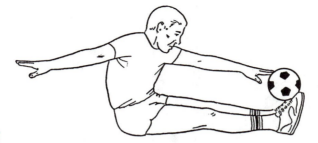

- No Great stretch
- Put Ball on altering
sides = more
torso

Figure 6-8. Seated stretch with ball.

Purpose: To stretch the muscles of the lower back and legs.

SP: Seated, holding a ball on the toes (instep) with one hand, legs extended or slightly flexed at the knee joint.

ES: Alternate hand position as shown, maintaining the ball position as illustrated.

Alter knee angle and
point toes to vary
stretch

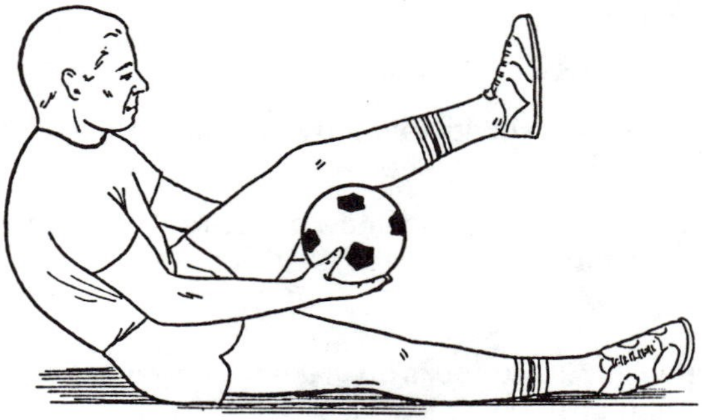

Figure 6-9. Seated figure-8 ball movement under the legs.

Purpose: To stretch the muscles of the lower back and legs.

SP: Seated, holding a ball, with the legs extended.

ES: Alternately raising one leg off the ground and then the other, move the ball under the leg from one hand to the other.

Note: Caution participants to avoid breath-holding during this exercise.

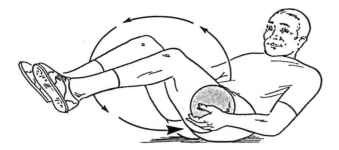

Figure 6-10. Leg circling clockwise and counterclockwise.

Purpose: To improve abdominal muscle tone.

SP: Sitting position.

ES: Lean rearward, lift heels off floor, and rotate the ball clockwise around the legs, then counterclockwise.

No breathing - common BREATHE!

Balance = Problem
Some shouldn't hold legs this long.
More hip flexion
↑MVO₂ w/o O₂ in - holding breath

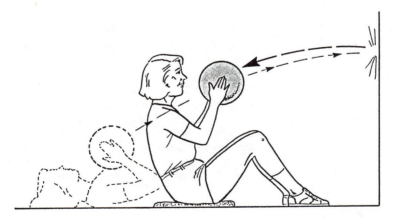

Figure 6-11. Sit-up-ball catching.

Purpose: To develop abdominal muscle tone.

SP: Lying position on a mat, at a distance of 3 to 4 feet from a wall, legs flexed at the knee joint.

ES: Push the ball to the wall with both hands and catch it on the rebound. As abdominal muscle strength improves, sit up and catch the ball.

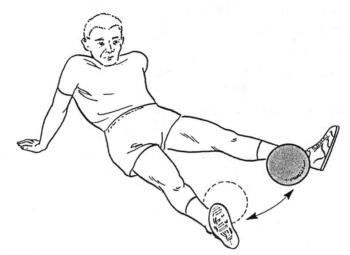

Figure 6-12. Leg squeeze.

Purpose: To tone the muscles of lower limbs and abdomen.

SP: Sitting with feet apart and legs extended at the knee joint, ball at left ankle.

ES: Lift legs off the ground and tap ball from left leg to right leg and back.

Note: Activity can be modified by squeezing the ball between the ankles and lifting the legs. This can be started with legs flexed at the knee joint and progressed to extended legs. It can also be used in a group circle relay, by passing the ball between the ankles from one person to another by rotating on the seat. However, participants should be cautioned to avoid breath-holding and excessive straining during the movement.

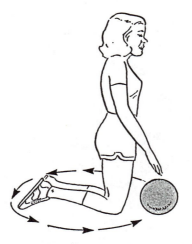

Figure 6-13. Ball circle around body in kneeling position.

Purpose: To stretch and exercise trunk rotator and anterior thigh muscles.

SP: Kneeling position on a mat with a ball placed on the mat surface.

ES: Using one or two hands and finger tip control, circle ball clockwise or counterclockwise around the body.

Prob.
Back Hurts
Tight Hams
Cardiaco
Older People

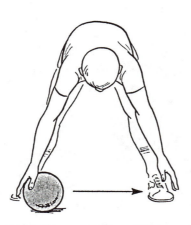

- Come up slowly
- Keep both hands on the ball
- Vary stance

Figure 6-14. Side-to-side ball movement on floor.

Purpose: To stretch the muscles of the lower back, arms, shoulders, and legs.

SP: Stand with the feet at shoulder width or wider, legs slightly flexed, leaning forward at the waist.

ES: Move the ball on the floor, side-to-side, between the feet.

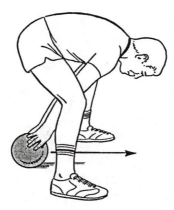

Figure 6-15. Forward-backward ball roll on floor.

Purpose: To stretch the muscles of the lower back, arms, shoulders, and legs.

SP: Stand with feet at shoulder width or wider, legs slightly flexed, leaning forward at the waist.

ES: Move the ball on the floor forward and backward between the feet.

Note: Try to move the ball at least 6 to 12 inches behind the heels.

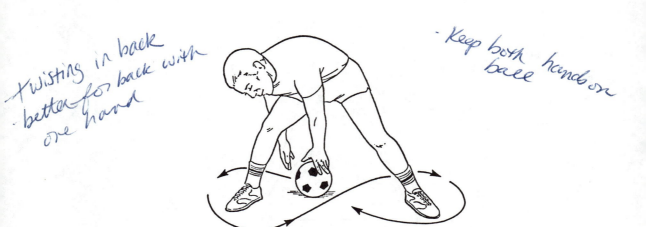

- twisting in back better for back with one hand

- Keep both hands on ball

Figure 6-16. Figure-8 ball movement on floor.

Purpose: To stretch the muscles of the lower back and legs.

SP: Stand with feet wide apart, legs slightly flexed at the knee joint, leaning forward at the waist.

ES: Move the ball with the hands in a figure-8 position around and between the feet. Ball should remain on the floor.

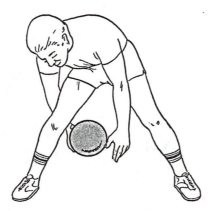

Figure 6-17. Figure-8 ball movement in air (off floor).

Purpose: To stretch the muscles of the lower back and legs.

SP: Stand with feet wide apart, legs slightly flexed at the knee joint, leaning forward at the waist.

ES: Move the ball with the hands in a figure-8 position around and between the legs. Ball should remain in the air.

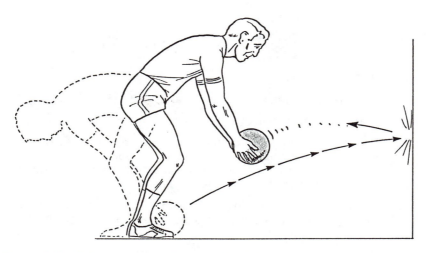

Figure 6-18. Ball centering wall rebound catch.

Purpose: To practice an agility move that requires timing and reaction.

SP: Football centering position with the ball on the floor, arms extended, legs flexed at shoulder width and the head slightly flexed, standing at a distance of 6 to 8 feet from the wall.

ES: Center the ball with two hands to the wall and quickly pivot 180 degrees and catch the rebounded ball on the fly. Alternate pivoting left and right. Vary distance to the wall.

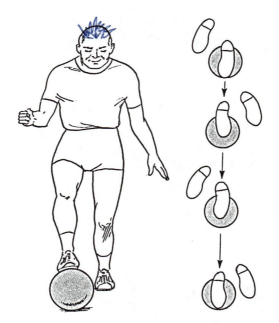

Figure 6-19. Foot-ball tapping.

Purpose: To gradually increase the heart rate and practice balance and agility.

SP: Standing with the ball of one foot resting on top of the ball.

ES: Tap the ball with the foot and alternate left and right legs. Start slowly and increase the tempo of ball tapping in a rhythmical manner. When skill is acquired, the ball can be moved a short distance forward and backward, left and right.

Note: Emphasize the maximum weight distribution on the support leg. The foot tap should not contribute to the balance of the participant.

- ↑HR rapidly
- risks of injury - esp. w/ age
- No breathing - need to!

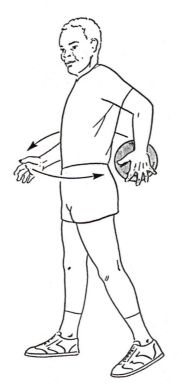

Figure 6-20. Ball rotation around waist.

Purpose: To stretch the muscles of the arms and shoulders.

SP: Stand, holding a ball at waist height.

ES: Rotate ball around the waist as shown, changing the direction occasionally with the hands.

Note: This activity can also be performed while the participant is walking, to gradually raise the heart rate.

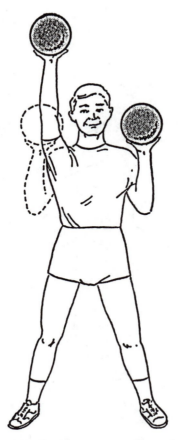

Figure 6-21. Arm-shoulder flexion and extension with two balls.

Purpose: To improve arm-shoulder mobility.

SP: Standing with hand held sport balls at shoulder height. Legs slightly wider than shoulder width.

ES: Alternate extending and flexing the arms (vertically upward) in a piston-like movement. Speed can be altered and a variety of sport balls can be used to include medicine balls of 2, 4, or 6 pounds.

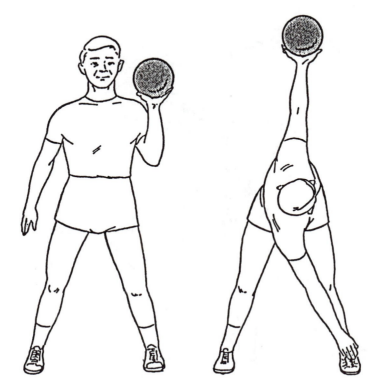

Figure 6-22. Trunk rotation with toe touching.

OK

Purpose: To increase trunk rotation range of motion and to practice balancing objects.

SP: Standing position with legs slightly wider than shoulder width. Feet are pointed straight ahead or toed inward.

ES: Extend the ball vertically upward with the left arm while simultaneously rotating the trunk to the left and touching the toe, ankle, or leg with the right hand. The head and eyes follow the hand held ball. Return to the starting position. Move the ball to the opposite hand and repeat the exercise. Slight flexion at the knee may be necessary.

- Ball size
- Problems:

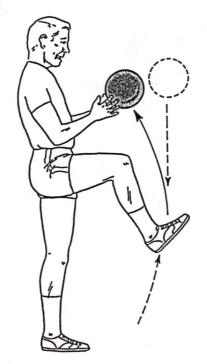

Figure 6-23. Foot-ball kick.

Purpose: To develop hand-eye-foot coordination and encourage hip flexion activity.

SP: Stand, holding a ball with the outstretched arms at shoulder height.

ES: Ball is dropped to knee level and kicked back and caught. Participant flexes the foot at the ankle joint for control. Alternate kicking legs.

Note: This activity can be performed while walking or jogging using the following sequences: 1-2-3 kick-catch, or, 1-2-3 kick with opposite leg and catch. The emphasis here should be on posture and ball control.

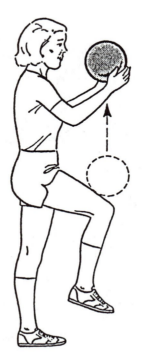

Figure 6-24. Thigh kick.

OR Purpose: To improve hand-eye coordination and increase hip flexion.

     SP: Stand, holding a ball at shoulder height.

     ES: Ball is dropped to hip level, rebounded with the thigh, and caught. Alternate right and left legs.

     Note: This stationary activity can be modified for rapid walking or jogging, using a 1-2-3 kick-catch sequence, alternating right and left thigh kicks. The emphasis should be on posture and ball control.

- Not good for elderly

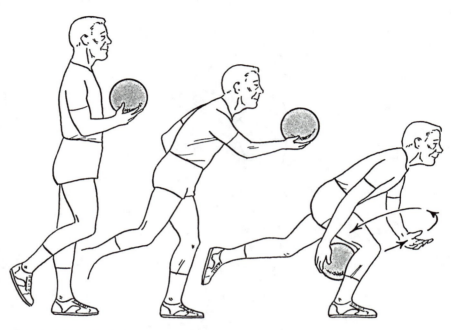

Figure 6-25. Ball balancing activity.

Purpose: To practice movements of static and dynamic balance.

SP: Standing on one foot with the ball held in a flexed arm position.

ES: Participant extends the arm of the hand held ball while flexing the leg at the knee joint. Non-support leg is extended (off the ground) to the rear. When a balanced position is achieved, the ball is circled about the support leg.

Sugges-
tions: Vary the degree of flexion of the support leg or non-support leg. Change support legs. Circle the ball at the ankle or waist. Close eyes during movement. Vary the size and weight of the ball.

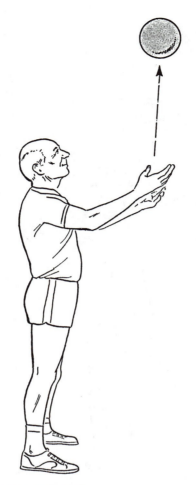

Figure 6-26. In front toss and catch.

Purpose: To gradually increase heart rate.

SP: Stand with the ball in both hands in front of body.

ES: Toss ball into air and catch (progress to walking and catching).

Note: Progress to walking and catching or to jogging and catching. This activity can also be modified to include a partner or more than one partner.

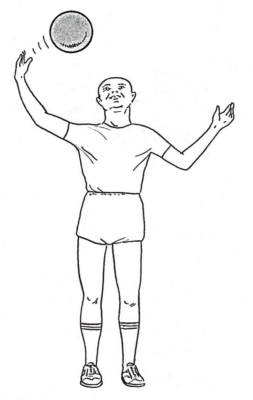

Figure 6-27. Air ball passing.

Purpose: To provide a low intensity warm-up activity and promote arm and shoulder flexibility.

SP: Standing, walking, or jogging.

ES: Ball is passed to opposite hand in arcs of varying heights while standing or in motion.

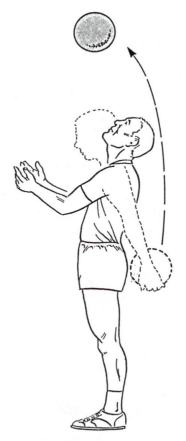

Figure 6-28. Behind-the-back ball flick and catch.

Purpose: To stretch muscles of arms, shoulders, lower back; to improve hand-eye coordination; to gradually increase heart rate.

SP: Stand with ball held in both hands behind back.

ES: Flick the ball up and over the head to be caught in front.

Note: Progress to walking and catching.

Note: Progress to flicking ball to a partner.

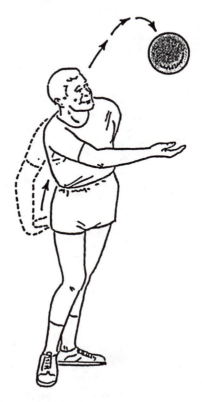

Figure 6-29. Same hand toss-and-catch.

Purpose: To stretch the muscles of the arms and shoulders and improve hand-eye coordination.

SP: Stand with one arm extended behind the back, below the waist, holding a ball.

ES: Toss the ball over the opposite shoulder (e.g., right hand tosses the ball forward, over the left shoulder) and catch it in front of the body with the same hand that tossed it.

Note: This activity can be modified by catching the ball with the opposite hand (i.e., right hand tosses the ball and the left hand catches it, or vice versa).

- can twist back / neck

Modification:
- toss with one hand & catch with both

80   *ON THE BALL*

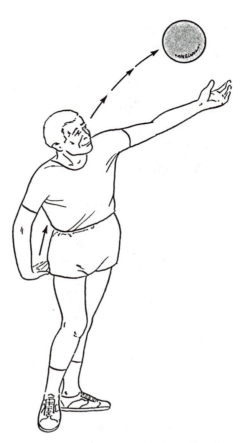

Figure 6-30. Ball passing behind back; standing or jogging.

Purpose: To develop hand-eye coordination and increase flexibility.

SP: Standing, holding a ball in one hand behind the buttocks.

ES: Toss the ball behind the back and catch with opposite hand. Alternate arms. As skill progresses, activity can be done while jogging.

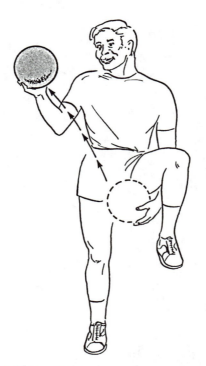

Figure 6-31. Ball passing under leg; standing or jogging.

Purpose: Increase range of motion of the leg and hip flexor muscles.

SP: Standing, holding a ball.

ES: Pass the ball under the flexed leg and catch with opposite hand. When jogging, a slight hop on the opposite leg is helpful for balance.

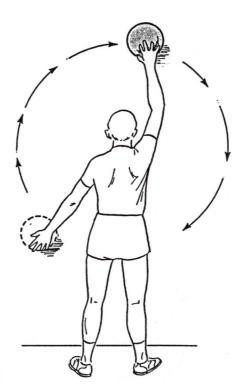

Figure 6-32. Arm circle with ball against wall.

OK Purpose: To stretch the muscles of the arms and shoulders.

SP: Stand facing a wall about 12 inches away, with the feet apart, holding a playground ball at waist height so that it rests between the outstretched hand and the wall.

ES: Move the ball in a full circle against the wall (i.e., left to right), changing hands when the ball is directly overhead. Alternately, move ball in the opposite direction (i.e., right to left) until several circles are completed.

Problems:
Arthritic

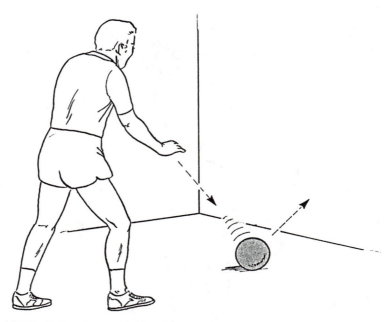

Figure 6-33. Ball volley against wall.

Purpose: To improve hand-eye coordination and gradually increase the heart rate. A good lead-up activity.

SP: Standing about 6 to 8 feet from a wall, holding a sport ball.

ES: Strike the ball with the palm or fist against the floor so that it rebounds off the adjacent wall, and strike again.

Note: Participants can be instructed to use either the right hand, left hand, or alternate hands.

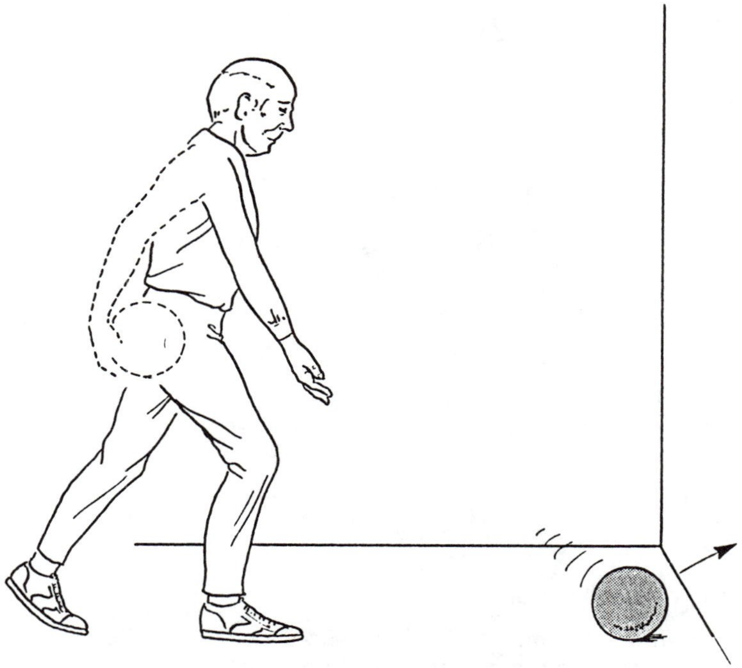

Figure 6-34. Bounce ball to wall.

Purpose: To stretch the muscles of arms and shoulders, and gradually increase the heart rate. A good lead-up activity.

SP: Ball in right hand, standing about 6 to 8 feet from a wall.

ES: Bounce ball from ground to wall and catch rebound.

Note: Toss and catch with: 1) right hand, 2) left hand, 3) both hands.

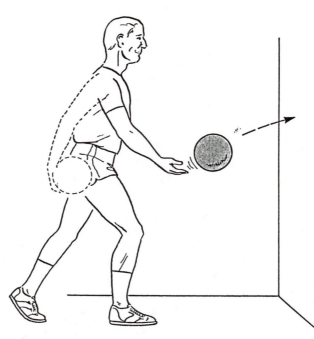

Figure 6-35. Toss ball to wall.

Purpose: To stretch the muscles of arms and shoulders, and gradually increase the heart rate. A good lead-up activity.

SP: Ball in right hand, standing about 6 to 8 feet from a wall.

ES: Toss ball to wall and catch rebound.

Note: Toss and catch with: 1) right hand, 2) left hand, 3) both hands. This
activity can also be done with a partner.

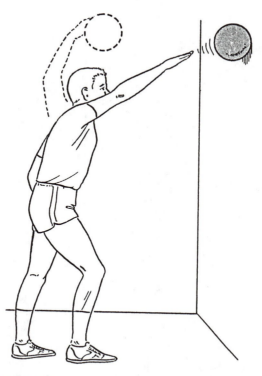

Figure 6-36. Swing and catch.

Purpose: To stretch the muscles of the arms and shoulders and gradually increase the heart rate. A good lead-up activity.

SP: Standing about 4 to 6 feet from a wall, holding a sport ball as illustrated.

ES: With the arm extended at the elbow joint, bounce the ball off wall to
catch and repeat.

Note: This activity can be performed with the right hand, the left hand, or
with a partner.

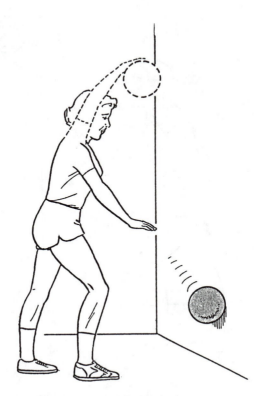

Figure 6-37. Swing and bounce to catch.

Purpose: To stretch the muscles of the arms and shoulders and gradually increase the heart rate. A good lead-up activity.

SP: Standing about 4 to 6 feet from a wall, holding a sport ball as illustrated.

ES: With an extended arm, bounce the ball off wall and ground to catch
and repeat.

Note: This activity can be performed with the right hand, the left hand, or
with a partner.

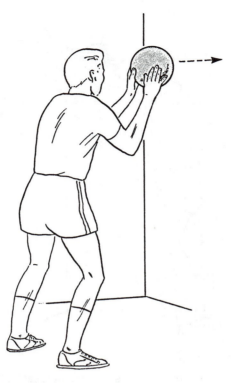

Figure 6-38. Push ball to wall.

Purpose: To stretch the muscles of the arms and shoulders and gradually increase the heart rate. A good lead-up activity.

SP: Standing about 5 to 6 feet from a wall, holding a sport ball at eye level.

ES: Extend arms to push ball to wall and catch.

Note: This activity can also be performed as a relay, or with a partner.

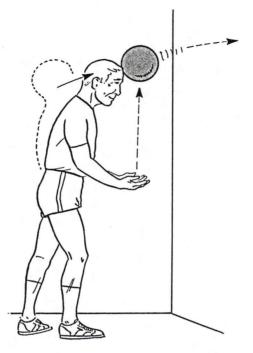

Figure 6-39. Head ball to wall.

Purpose: To gradually increase the heart rate; an ideal lead-up activity.

SP: Stand 3 to 4 feet from a wall, holding a ball.

ES: Toss ball into air, strike it with the forehead on to the wall and catch. Repeat.

Note: This activity can also be performed with a partner, or adapted to a relay. One person tosses the ball to a wall and it is then headed on the rebound by the other.

7

Partner Stationary Activities

The following partner exercises, using a playground ball, volleyball, or other sports equipment, are primarily designed for the stretching portion of the warm-up and cool-down. For all exercises: Purpose = primary reason for activity and/or focus on muscle groups that are employed; SP = starting position; ES = exercise sequence; and, Note = special considerations and/or modifications.

The number of repetitions of each activity or time allotted for them is left to the exercise leader's discretion.

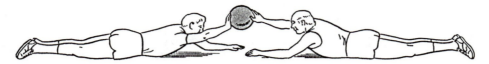

Figure 7-1. Partner shoulder stretch with ball in the prone position.

Purpose: To stretch the muscles of the arms, shoulders, and lower back.

SP: Lying on the floor, facing partner, one hand on the ground, the other hand holding a ball in mid-air, 6 to 8 inches above the ground.

ES: Lower the ball to the ground, change hands, and lift ball again to starting position. Both partners should use the *same* hand (i.e., either both right, or both left) when holding the ball in mid-air.

Note: Caution participants to avoid breath-holding during the exercise.

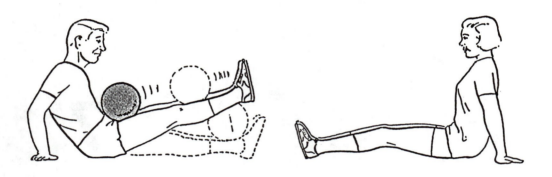

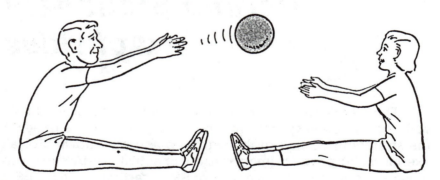

Figure 7-2. Seated ball-leg-roll with partner.

Purpose: To stretch and tone muscles of the abdomen.

SP: Seated, legs extended, feet together and dorsiflexed, ball balanced in anterior portion of lower legs and feet.

ES: Elevate extended legs and allow ball to roll to abdomen. Pick ball up and toss to partner. Reverse roles.

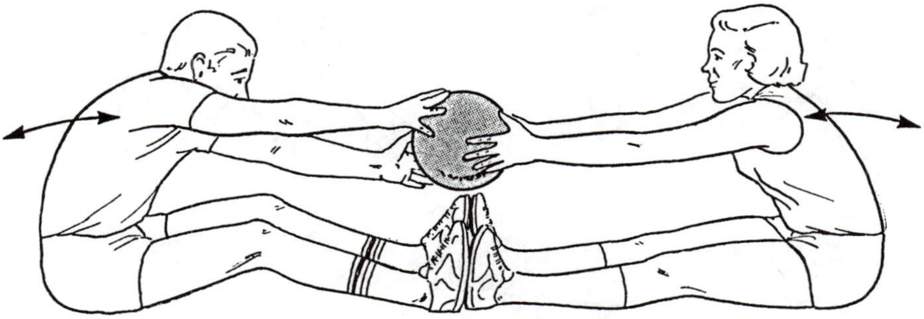

Figure 7-3. Partner stretch with ball.

Purpose: To stretch the muscles of the arms, shoulders, lower back, and legs.

SP: Seated, facing a partner, feet against feet, legs flat on the floor or slightly flexed at the knee joint.

ES: Pass the ball with the hands from one partner to another, leaning forward as the ball is exchanged.

Note: This exercise can be modified to a "static stretch" with both partners holding the ball simultaneously over the feet and maintaining this position for 10 seconds.

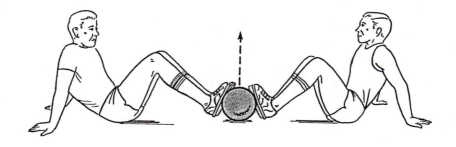

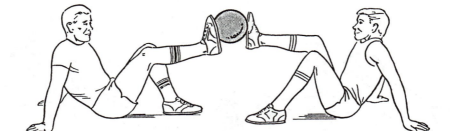

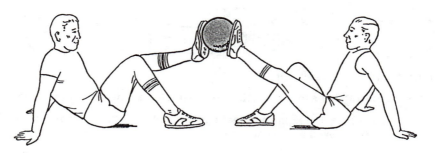

Figure 7-4. Ball suspension with partner.

Purpose: To stretch and tone the muscles of the abdomen.

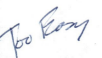

SP: Seated, facing partner, hands on the floor for support, both legs flexed, with a ball held in the air between partner's feet.

ES: Alternate feet so as to maintain ball in mid-air position. Both partners should use the *same* leg (i.e., either both right, or both left) when supporting the ball in mid-air.

Note: Emphasize that both legs of both partners should be flexed throughout the exercise, that one foot of each partner should *always* be on the floor, and that breath-holding should be avoided.

Note: This activity can be made even more challenging by having the exercise leader walking among the pairs of participants, tossing a separate sport ball. The ball is caught, while simultaneously maintaining another ball in mid-air position with a partner, and thrown back to the leader.

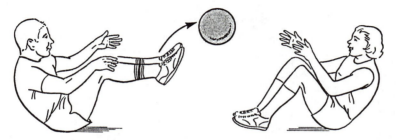

Figure 7-5. Seated ball-leg-flick with partner.

Purpose: To stretch and tone the muscles of the abdomen.

SP: Seated, facing a partner, legs flexed at the knee joint, feet together.

ES: One partner places the ball on the legs at the level of the knees and allows it to roll down the legs toward the feet. As the ball approaches the ankle the feet are suddenly raised off the floor, "flicking" the ball in the air to the other partner who catches it and repeats the sequence.

No tone to Abs

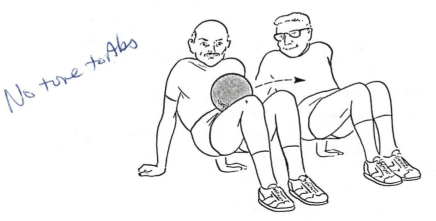

Figure 7-6. Bridge ball.

Purpose: Tone muscles of the abdomen and gradually increase heart rate (see note).

SP: Sit on ground with legs flexed, ball on the abdomen, with partner's shoulders and hips almost touching.

ES: Lift buttocks to form a "bridge" and pass ball from one partner's abdomen to other partner's abdomen without touching ball with hands.

Note: Person with ball can move forwards, backwards, sideways left or right, with partner following or staying in position. This activity can also be adapted to a "line" or "circle" relay format.

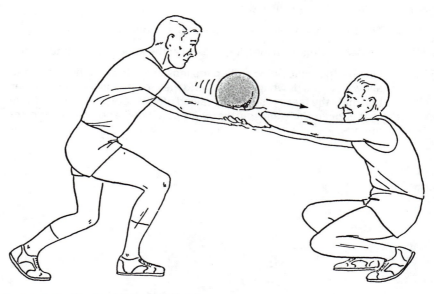

Figure 7-7. Squat with arm-ball roll.

Purpose: To tone the muscles of the abdomen and lower limbs.

SP: Clasp wrists as shown, balance ball between arms and stand upright.

ES: Alternate squatting and standing upright, keep the ball rolling on the arms.

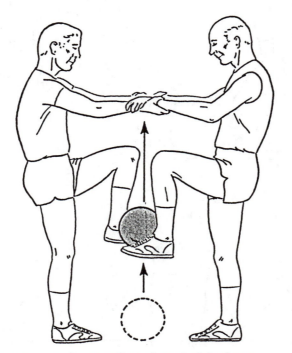

Figure 7-8. Ball lift with feet to partners' outstretched arms.

Purpose: To improve balance, flexibility and coordination. (This serves as an ideal activity to "challenge" participants at the end of an exercise session.)

SP: Stand, facing a partner, wrists locked as shown, with a playground ball on the floor.

ES: Partners simultaneously move their feet to the sides of the ball so that it can be lifted, straight up, with the medial portion of their ankles, to the outstretched arms which grasp it between the wrists. Each partner must use the same leg (i.e., right to right or left to left) when lifting the ball, slowly flexing the knee as the ball is raised.

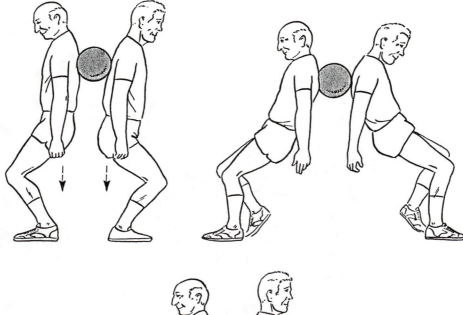

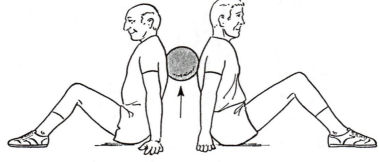

Cant Do
: Too Hard

No good
for knees

Figure 7-9. Sit back-to-back with ball.

Purpose: To tone the abdominal muscles and muscles of lower limbs.

SP: Stand upright, back-to-back, with ball between backs.

ES: Flex legs, moving down slowly to sit, then stand up keeping ball be-
         tween backs at all times.

Note: This basic exercise of sitting down and standing up can be done with
         the ball in various positions between partners (e.g., hip-to-hip,
         shoulder-to-shoulder.)

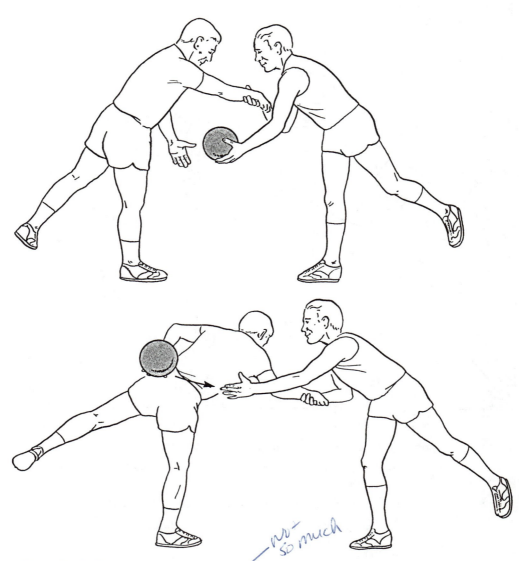

Figure 7-10. Partner balance with ball exchange.

Purpose: To enhance balance, flexibility, and coordination.

SP: Stand, facing partner, lock wrists, and balance on one leg while the other leg is extended rearward.

ES: Hand the ball back and forth, under the locked wrists, over the locked wrists, behind the back, or under the non-support leg.

Note: The exercise leader should emphasize creativity during this activity.

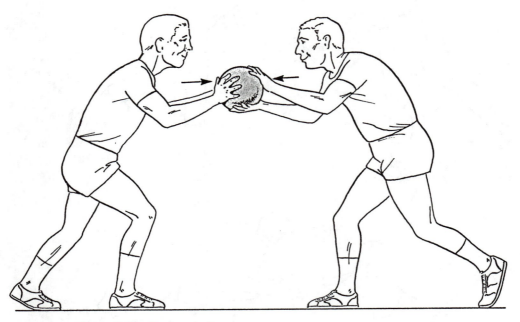

Figure 7-11. Push-o-ball.

Purpose: To tone the muscles of the upper limbs, trunk, and lower limbs.

SP: Partners hold the ball (as shown) but with arms slightly flexed at the elbow joint.

ES: Each partner resists being pushed back by the other.

Note: Caution participants to avoid breath holding.

No to Candice

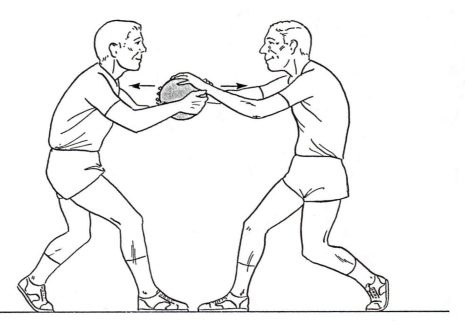

Figure 7–12. Tug-o-ball.

Purpose: To tone the muscles of the upper limbs, trunk and lower limbs.

SP: Partners hold ball (as shown) but with arms slightly flexed at the elbow joint.

ES: Each partner resists being pulled forward by the other.

Note: Breath-holding and excessive straining should be avoided during this activity.

Not Cardiac

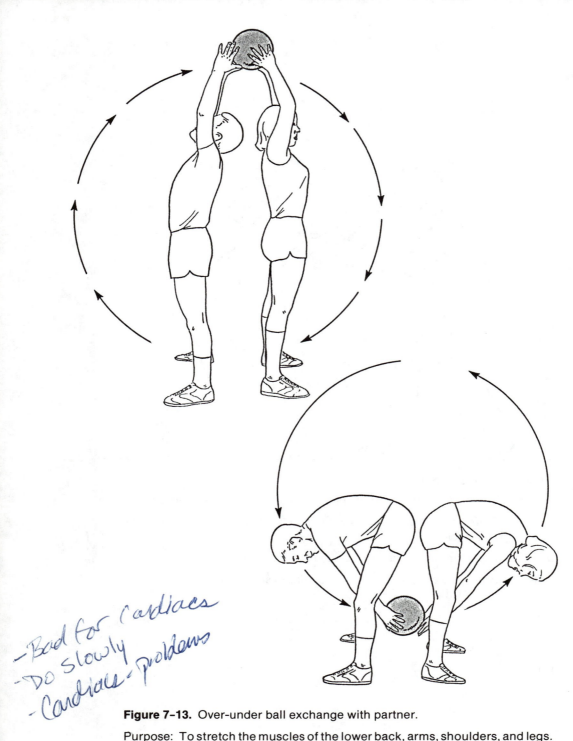

- Bad for cardiacs
- Do slowly
- Cardiac problems

Figure 7–13. Over-under ball exchange with partner.

Purpose: To stretch the muscles of the lower back, arms, shoulders, and legs.

SP: Standing, back-to-back, about 2 feet from partner.

ES: Hand the ball over the head (arms extended) and between the legs as shown. Repeat sequence several times.

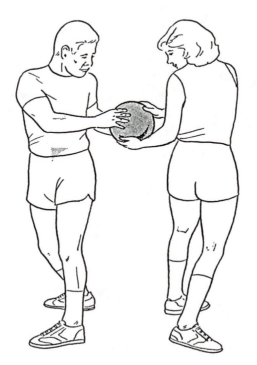

Figure 7-14. Side twist with partner.

Purpose: To stretch the muscles of the arms, shoulders, abdomen, and trunk.

SP: Standing, back-to-back, about 2 feet from a partner. One individual is holding a ball. Feet are pointed forward.

ES: Both partners rotate in the same direction (e.g., both to the left), so that the ball can be exchanged as shown. The partners now rotate in the opposite direction (e.g., both to the right) and the ball is handed off again.

Note: The feet should remain flat on the floor during the entire exercise sequence. There should be slight flexion at the knee joint to encourage increased range of motion.

Trunk exp.
- Control temps

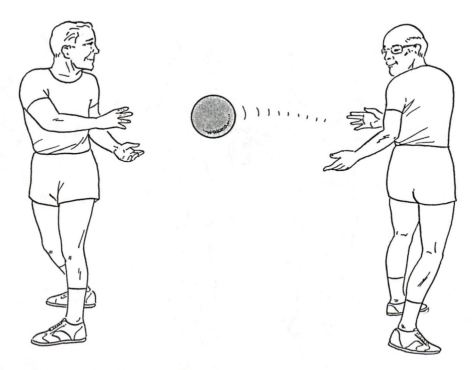

Figure 7–15. Side twist and ball toss with partner.

Purpose: To stretch the muscles of the abdomen and trunk.

SP: Standing, back-to-back, at least 5 feet from a partner, with feet pointed forward, hip width apart.

ES: Rotate in same direction as partner (i.e., both right or both left) and toss ball to partner.

Note: The feet should remain flat on the floor during the entire exercise sequence.

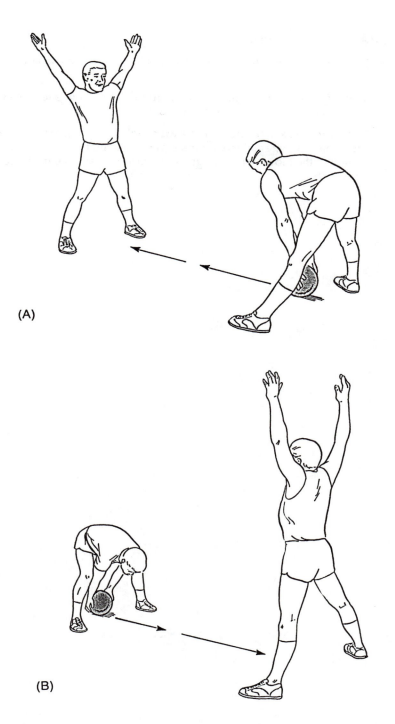

(A)

(B)

Figure 7-16. Forward ball roll to partner. See legend on page 106 for explanation.

Figure 7-16. Forward ball roll to partner.

Purpose: To stretch the muscles of the arms, shoulders, lower back, and abdomen.

SP: Stand, facing partner, approximately 10 to 15 feet from each other, feet spread apart and pointed forward.

ES: One partner flexes the trunk at the waist, rolls ball on ground to opposite partner, stretching with the arms above the head at the conclusion of the movement (A). The other partner then repeats the sequence (B).

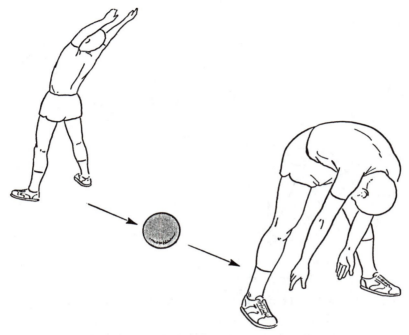

Figure 7–17. Backward ball roll to partner.

Purpose: To stretch muscles of the arms, shoulders, lower back, and abdomen.

SP: Stand, partners facing opposite directions, approximately 10 to 15 feet from each other, feet spread apart and pointed forward.

ES: One partner flexes the trunk at the waist, rolls ball on ground (between legs) to opposite partner, standing up and stretching with the arms above the head at the conclusion of the movement. The person receiving the ball bends forward, looking between the legs and behind, and the sequence is repeated. In essence, one partner is always bending forward while the other is standing upright, and vice versa.

Note: Since the partners cannot initially see the ball rolling toward them, this activity requires precise timing and coordination. Using verbal cues as "now" or the person's name is encouraged.

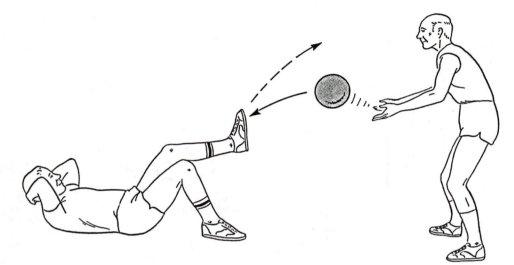

Figure 7-18. Ball kick with partner.

Purpose: To stretch and tone the muscles of the legs and abdomen.

SP: One person lies on his back, placing one foot on the floor (knee flexed), while the other leg and foot are raised. A partner stands 4 to 6 feet from him, holding a ball.

ES: The partner standing tosses the ball *underhand* toward the raised foot of the partner on the ground. The partner on the ground taps the ball back to the standing partner, alternating feet. After several repetitions, the partners reverse positions.

Note: This activity can also be performed with both legs raised simultaneously, feet together, having the lower back in contact with the floor.

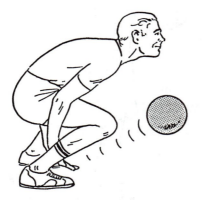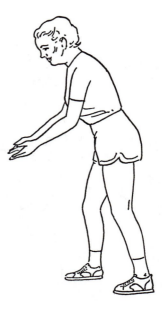

Figure 7-19. Ball 'flick' to partner.

Purpose: To stretch the muscles of the lower back, abdomen, arms, and legs. (NOTE: This activity requires a considerable amount of dexterity and may be too difficult for some individuals.)

SP: Stand, facing a partner, about 6 to 8 feet apart. One of the participants has placed a playground ball on the floor between his feet which are shoulder width apart.

ES: The participant with the ball leans forward by slowly flexing the legs while simultaneously reaching down *behind* the legs to grasp the ball. The ball is then 'flicked' between his legs to the partner who catches it, and the roles are now reversed.

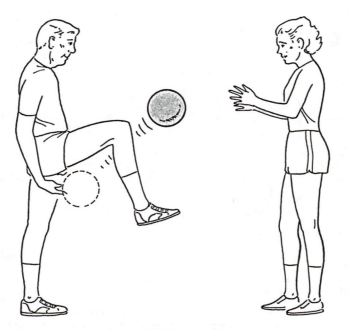

Figure 7-20. Ball toss under leg with partner.

Purpose: To improve coordination and stretch the hip flexor muscles.

SP: Stand, facing a partner, from 10 to 20 feet apart, with one person holding a playground ball.

ES: The partner holding the ball lifts a leg (with the knee flexed) and tosses the ball under it to the other partner who catches it. The roles are now reversed and the activity continues.

Note: This activity can be modified by alternating flexed legs and hand that is tossing the ball.

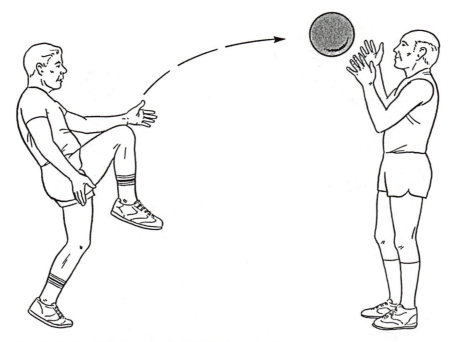

Figure 7–21. Ball drop, knee kick, with partner.

Purpose: To stretch and tone the muscles of the legs and abdomen.

SP: Stand, facing partner, about 5 to 10 feet apart, with one partner holding a ball at shoulder height.

ES: The ball is dropped close to the body and the leg is simultaneously raised, knee flexed, striking the ball on the front portion of the thigh to the opposite partner who catches it and repeats the sequence. The raised leg should be alternated by each partner.

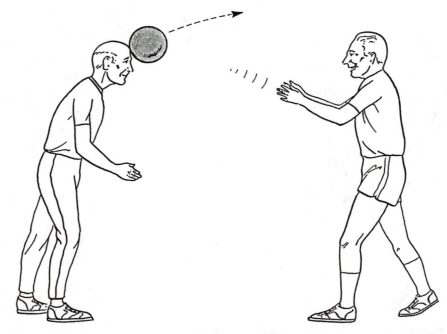

Figure 7-22. Ball heading using a light sport ball.

Purpose: To encourage low-intensity head control activity with an emphasis on timing.

SP: Partners face one another at a variable distance of 6 to 8 feet apart. One person is holding a ball.

ES: A two-hand under arm toss with a slight arc is made toward a partner. The partner heads the ball for a return catch. Variation: The person tossing the ball heads it himself, with the partner catching it.

Note: Avoid head flexion. Activity is contraindicated when subjects have cervical vertebrate problems or are wearing glasses.

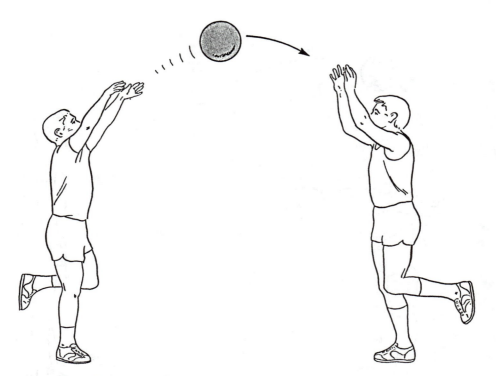

Figure 7-23. Ball toss with partner, alternating feet.

Purpose: To promote balance and agility and gradually raise the heart rate.

SP: Standing, facing a partner while balancing on one leg, one partner holding a ball.

ES: Toss the ball back and forth between partners while alternating the balancing leg with each toss.

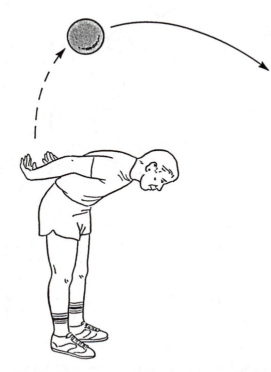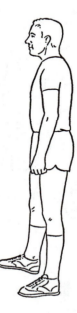

Figure 7-24. Behind-the-back ball toss to partner.

Purpose: To stretch the muscles of the arms, shoulders, lower back, and abdomen.

SP: Standing, facing a partner, about 10 to 15 feet apart, with one person holding a ball behind the back with both hands.

ES: The person holding the ball flexes the trunk forward quickly, "flicking" it to his partner who catches it and repeats the sequence.

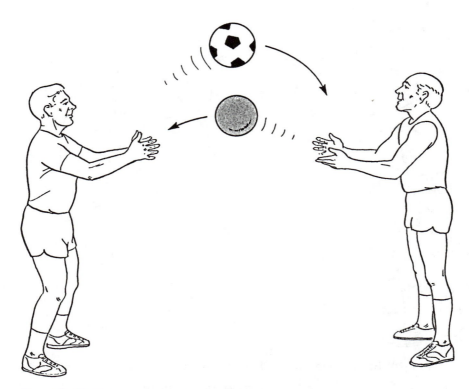

Figure 7-25. Ball juggling with partner.

Purpose: To enhance hand-eye coordination and agility.

SP: Stand about 8 to 12 feet from a partner, with each person holding a ball.

ES: Toss balls simultaneously, back and forth between partners, with one person tossing "high," and the other tossing "low," and then alternating "high - low."

Note: This is a "fun" activity that requires both coordination and concentration, particularly when partners alternate their tosses from "high" to "low." The exercise leader can turn this activity into a contest to see which pair can achieve the highest number of consecutive tosses, without dropping a ball. A floor bounce can also be incorporated. In addition, this activity can be performed while moving in a side slide or forward-rearward direction.

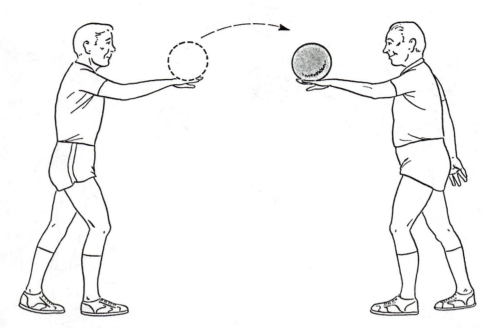

Figure 7–26. Back-of-the hand ball toss to partner.

Purpose: To improve hand-eye coordination and timing.

SP: Standing about 3 to 5 feet from a partner, facing each other, with one
          arm extended in front of the body at shoulder height, palm facing
          downward. One person has a sport ball balanced on the *back* of his
          hand.

ES: The individual with the ball tosses it to his partner, who catches it on
          the back of his hand. Roles are now reversed, and the activity is con-
          tinued.

Note: This activity can be made even more challenging by having individu-
          als walking, each balancing a sport ball on the back of the hand. As
          two participants approach each other, face to face, they concur-
          rently toss the balls in the air, attempting to catch the other person's
          ball on the back of the hand.

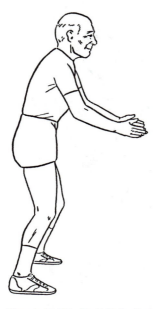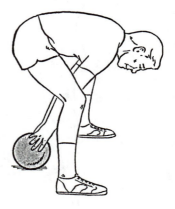

Figure 7-27. Ball "hike" to partner.

Purpose: To stretch muscles of the arms, shoulders, lower back, and abdomen.

SP: Stand, partners facing the same direction, approximately 10 to 15 feet from each other, with one person holding a playground ball.

ES: The partner with the ball leans forward and "hikes" it to the person behind, who catches it. Both individuals now turn to face the opposite direction and the activity is continued with the roles reversed.

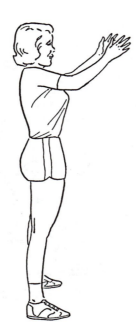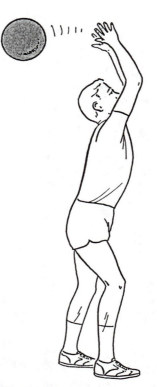

Figure 7-28. Backward overhead ball toss with partner.

Purpose: To stretch the muscles of the arms, shoulders, and torso and improve hand-eye coordination.

SP: Stand about 8 to 12 feet from a partner, with both individuals facing
the same direction. One partner is holding a ball.

ES: The partner with ball tosses it overhead and behind him while the
other individual catches it. Both partners then change direction and
reverse roles, and the sequence is repeated.

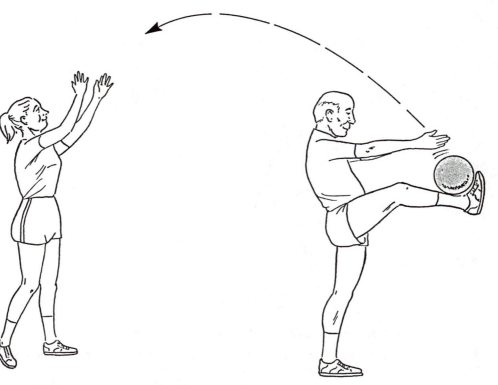

Figure 7-29. Ball kick overhead to partner.

Purpose: To increase hip flexion mobility and improve coordination.

SP: Standing, partners facing the same direction, approximately 15 to 20
         feet apart, with one person holding a playground ball.

ES: Forward participant drops a ball from shoulder height and kicks it
         overhead. Ball is kicked at hip-level height and the foot position is
         dorsiflexion. Participant to the rear catches the ball. Both individuals
         now turn to face the opposite direction and the activity is continued
         with the roles reversed.

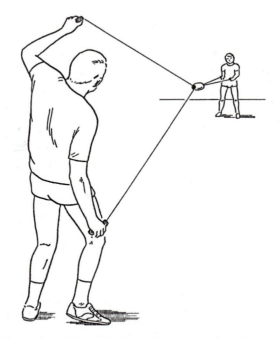

Figure 7–30. Operation of the Playbuoy® arm exerciser.*

Purpose: To strengthen and aerobically condition the upper body, improve coordination and timing, and have fun.

SP: The device includes a plastic buoy (similar to the standard swimming-pool lane-divider rope buoy) on two 20-foot waxed lines attached to 4 plastic handles. While standing, each partner grasps a pair of handles.

ES: During operation, the buoy is shuttled back and forth between 2 partners by alternating opening and closing of the handles. By changing the hand position, or the directional spread of the handles, different angles of pull can be attained to exercise varied upper body muscle groups.

*Originally described by Frost, G. The Playbuoy® exercise device. Amer. Corr. Ther. J. 31:156, 1977. (The Playbuoy® exercise device, Pat. No. 3,743,280, is available through Gilbert Sacks Inc., P.O. Box 4578, El Monte, California 91734.)

8

Individual Continuous Movement Activities

The following individual activities, using a playground ball or volleyball, are primarily designed for the cardiorespiratory portion of the warm-up or to complement the endurance phase. For all exercises: Purpose = primary reason for activity and/or focus on muscle groups that are employed; SP = starting position; ES = exercise sequence; and, Note = special considerations and/or modifications.

The number of repetitions of each activity or time allotted for them is left to the exercise leader's discretion.

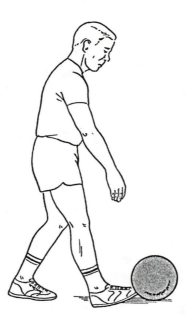

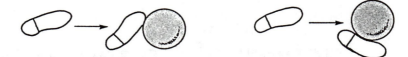

Figure 8-1. Foot-dribble around room.

Purpose: To gradually increase the heart rate.

SP: Standing with the ball on the floor in front of the feet.

ES: Tap the ball gently with the feet while walking around the outside of the room.

Note: Caution participants to move the ball only 2 or 3 feet with each kick, being careful to avoid tripping on it. The ball is struck using either the medial or lateral portions of the foot, the heel, or the toes.

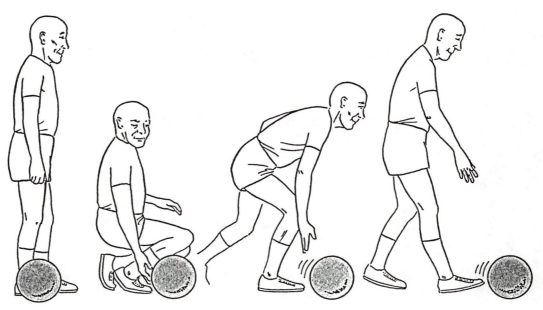

Figures 8–2. Controlled ball bowling exercise.

Purpose: To encourage postural changes and develop leg muscle endurance.

SP: Standing with ball adjacent to left or right foot.

ES: Stoop to a fixed leg position, back extended and head up and push the ball forward. Move to an upright position, walk or jog after ball and repeat the activity. Ball can be pushed by alternating left and right hands. Keep the velocity of the ball under control.

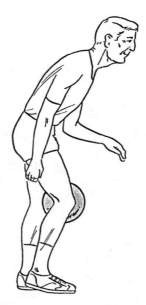

Figure 8–3. Knee shuffle walk.

Purpose: A movement pattern used to change the tempo of an aerobic exercise segment.

SP: Standing with the ball placed between the knees. Arms are relaxed and at the sides.

ES: Participant moves forward or backward using a shuffle gait to keep ball between the knees. Foot placement is forward with toes pointed slightly inward.

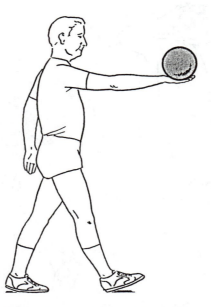

Figure 8–4. Back-of-the-hand ball balance while walking.

Purpose: To stretch the muscles of the arms and shoulders, improve hand-eye coordination, and gradually raise the heart rate.

SP: Stand with one arm outstretched, as shown, balancing a playground ball *on the back of the hand*.

ES: The participant begins walking while simultaneously maintaining the ball balanced on the back of the hand.

Note: The exercise leader can make the activity even more challenging (and enjoyable) by emphasizing that participants walk in varied directions. Thus, the participants will also have to employ peripheral vision to avoid colliding with each other.

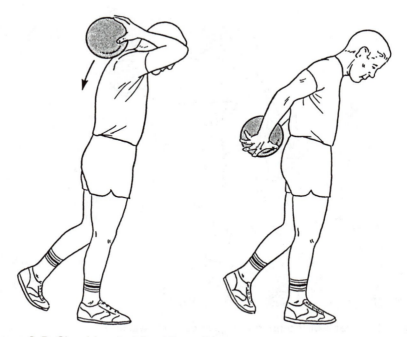

Figure 8–5. Shoulder stretch while walking.

Purpose: To stretch the muscles of the arms and shoulders while gradually raising the heart rate.

SP: Standing, while holding a ball with one hand on the curved part of the upper back, between the shoulder blades.

ES: While walking, release the ball so that it rolls down the back. Quickly move both hands to the position as shown, so as to catch the ball at the lower back (before it falls to the ground). Repeat the sequence.

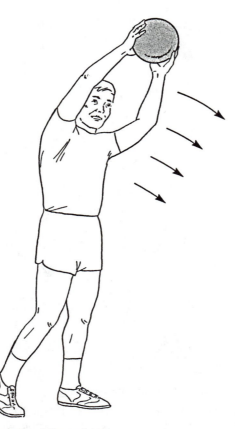

Figure 8-6. Side stretch while walking.

Purpose: To stretch the muscles of the abdomen and trunk and gradually raise the heart rate.

SP: Standing, arms outstretched with the ball held over the head.

ES: While walking briskly, gently flex the trunk from side to side while holding a ball overhead.

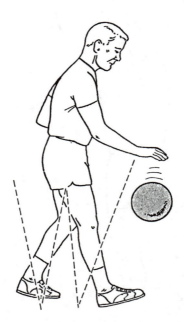

Figure 8-7. Low-ball dribble while slow walking.

Purpose: To gradually raise the heart rate and improve hand-eye coordination. Accordingly, this is an excellent aerobic warm-up activity.

SP: Stand with the feet apart, holding a playground ball.

ES: Start walking slowly, taking short strides while dribbling the ball rapidly so that it bounces to a height below waist level before it is struck with the hand again.

Note: This activity can be modified by alternating hands on each successive dribble. Individuals can also dribble while sidestepping, while walking backwards, or while moving forward and completing a 360-degree turn.

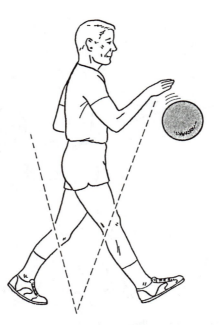

Figure 8–8. High-ball dribble while fast walking.

Purpose: To gradually raise the heart rate and improve hand-eye coordination. Accordingly, this is an excellent aerobic warm-up activity.

SP: Stand with the feet apart, holding a playground ball.

ES: Start walking briskly, taking long strides while dribbling the ball slowly so that it bounces to approximately shoulder height before it is struck with the hand again.

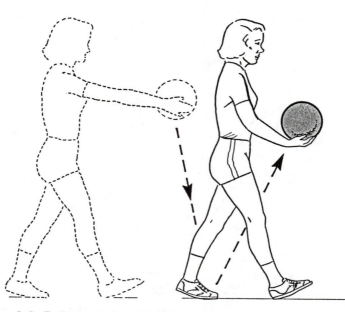

Figure 8-9. Ball toss and catch while walking.

Purpose: To stretch the muscles of the arms and shoulders, improve hand-eye coordination, and gradually raise the heart rate.

SP: Stand with the arms outstretched, holding a playground ball between the hands.

ES: Start walking briskly while simultaneously dropping the ball in front, *with backspin*, so that it can bounce off the floor and be caught, without breaking stride.

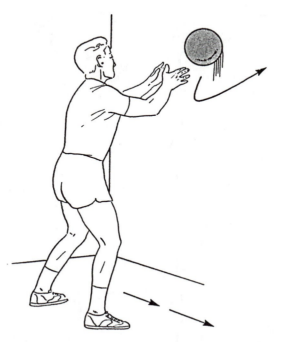

Figure 8-10. Ball bounce against wall while sidestepping.

Purpose: To promote agility and gradually raise the heart rate.

SP: Standing, facing a wall, feet apart, while holding a ball.

ES: Sidestepping or sidesliding around the circumference of a room, toss the ball against the walls and catch it, while moving continuously.

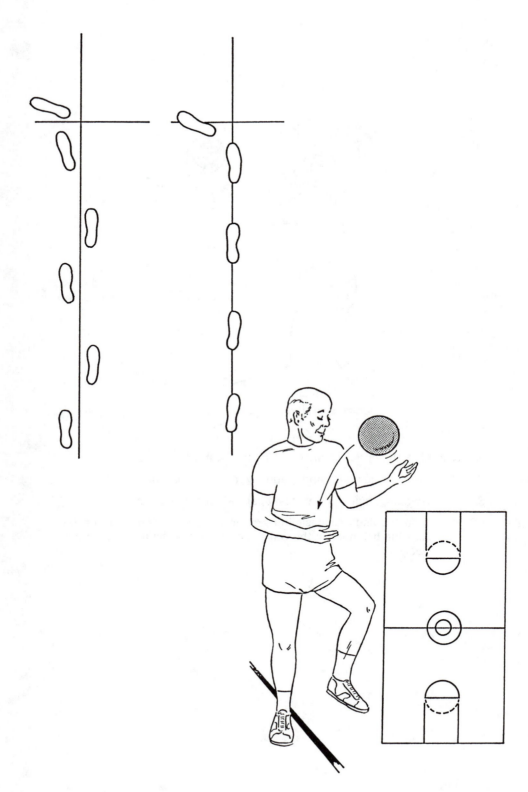

Figure 8–11. Floor line walking maneuvers.

Purpose: To improve balance and coordination and gradually raise the heart rate. (NOTE: This is an activity that is particularly applicable for the warm-up phase of the exercise session.)

SP: A large group of participants, each holding a playground ball, using a facility that has line demarcations for basketball.

ES: The exercise leader requests that the participants start walking in varied directions, either walking directly on any floor line or avoiding floor lines by stepping over them. The former activity can be challenging when two participants who are walking on the same line approach each other forcing one to leap to another line. These lines may be described as a "tightrope" by the exercise leader. The latter activity (i.e., avoiding floor lines by stepping over them) can be modified by the exercise leader who may suggest that each line represents a 6-, 12-, or 18-inch hurdle that must be leaped over by the participants who step higher and higher to "clear" these imaginary hurdles. Either activity can be performed with or without a playground ball. If a ball is employed, it can be simultaneously juggled from hand to hand, or moved around the waist while the participant walks on or steps over floor lines.

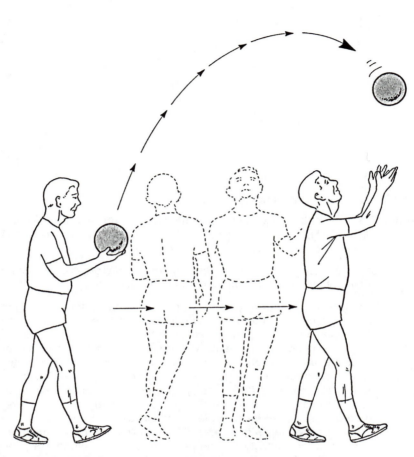

Figure 8-12. Ball catching after a 360-degree turn.

Purpose: To practice balance and orient to objects in space.

SP: Standing, holding a sport ball in front of the body at chest height.

ES: While walking, toss the ball up and forward in the air, complete a 360-degree turn clockwise or counterclockwise and catch the ball. As skill improves, move from a fast walk to jogging.

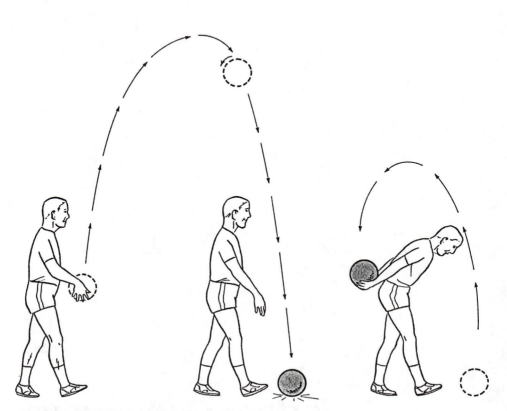

Figure 8-13. Ball toss with behind-the-back catch.

Purpose: To stretch the muscles of the upper arm, back and shoulders, improve coordination, and gradually increase the heart rate.

SP: While walking, hold the ball at waist height, as shown.

ES: Toss the ball out in front of the body *with backspin* at a height of at least 12 to 14 feet from the ground. Continue walking forward and, as the ball bounces off the floor, catch it behind the back with the outstretched arms and hands.

Notes: The participant should develop his/her coordination to perform this activity *while maintaining a steady walking pace* rather than stopping to catch the ball.

9

Partner Continuous Movement Activities

The following partner activities, using a playground ball or volleyball, are primarily designed for the cardiorespiratory portion of the warm-up or to complement the endurance phase. For all exercises: Purpose = primary reason for activity and/or focus on muscle groups that are employed; SP = starting position; ES = exercise sequence; and, Note = special considerations and/or modifications.

The number of repetitions of each activity or time allotted for them is left to the exercise leader's discretion.

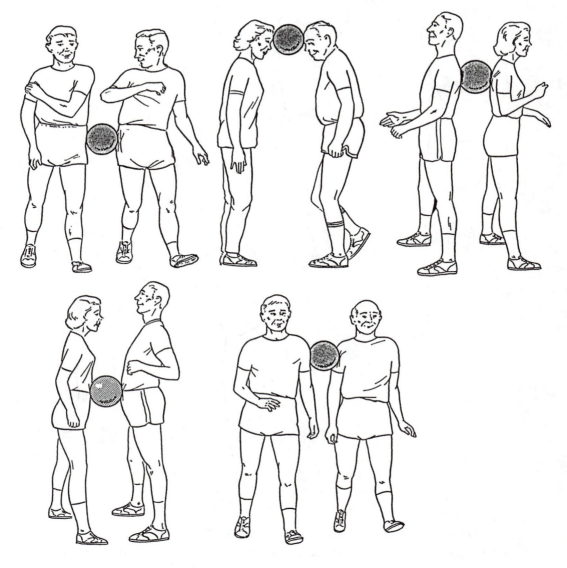

Figure 9-1. Ball kept between partners.

Purpose: To gradually increase heart rate.

SP: Stand upright with ball between partners.

ES: Move forwards, backwards, to left or to right on command, keeping ball in position.

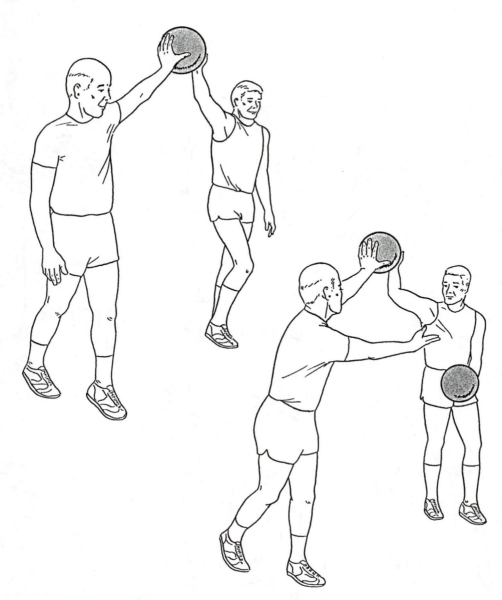

Figure 9–2. Ball support with partner while walking.

Purpose: To stretch the arm and shoulder muscles and gradually raise the heart rate.

SP: Standing, side-by-side with a partner, with a ball held between partners as illustrated.

ES: Walk around the room while maintaining this position.

Note: This activity can be modified by tossing another ball with the outside arm between partners.

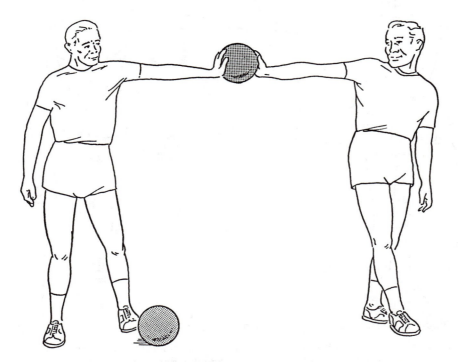

Figure 9–3. Ball suspension and foot dribble with partner while walking.

Purpose: To stretch the muscles of the arms and shoulders and gradually raise the heart rate.

SP: Standing, partners facing the same direction, about 4 to 6 feet from each other, supporting a playground ball at shoulder height with the inside hand (elbows slightly flexed). One partner has a second ball on the floor near his feet.

ES: As the partners begin walking around, maintaining one ball supported between them at shoulder height, the second ball is foot dribbled back and forth (i.e., from one partner to another).

Note: Participants should be cautioned to gently foot dribble the ball and keep it under control. This will prevent tripping on the ball.

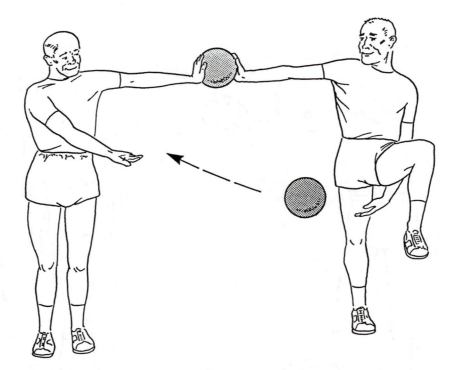

Figure 9-4. Ball suspension and toss with partner while walking.

Purpose: To stretch the muscles of the arms, shoulders and legs, improve hand-eye coordination, and gradually increase the heart rate.

SP: Standing, partners facing the same direction, about 4 to 6 feet from each other, supporting a playground ball at shoulder height with the inside hand (elbows slightly flexed). One partner is holding a second playground ball.

ES: As the partners begin walking around the floor, maintaining one ball supported between them, the second ball is tossed under an outstretched leg from one individual to another who catches it. The objective of the activity is to maintain the walking pace even when the ball is tossed from one partner to another. Variations include tossing the ball under the inside leg and changing ball support arms upon command.

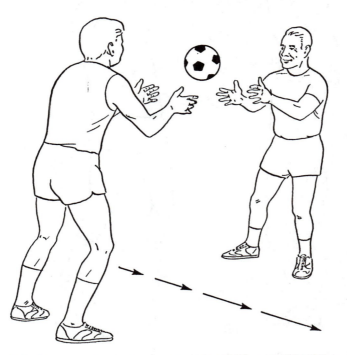

Figure 9-5. Ball toss with partner while sidestepping or sidesliding.

Purpose: To promote lateral agility and gradually raise the heart rate.

SP: Standing, while facing a partner, with one partner holding a ball.

ES: While slowly sidestepping across the floor, toss the ball back and forth between partners.

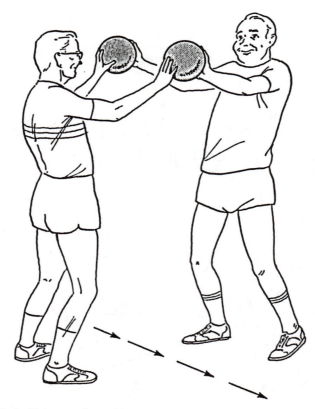

Figure 9–6. Sidestepping with partner.

Purpose: To stretch the muscles of the arms and shoulders and gradually raise the heart rate.

SP: Standing, facing a partner, about 3 to 4 feet apart, arms outstretched, with each hand supporting a ball as shown.

ES: Sidestep with partner in one direction or another while maintaining balls at shoulder level.

Note: This activity can be modified by having the participants move forwards, backwards, to the left or to the right, or doing 360-degree rotations on command.

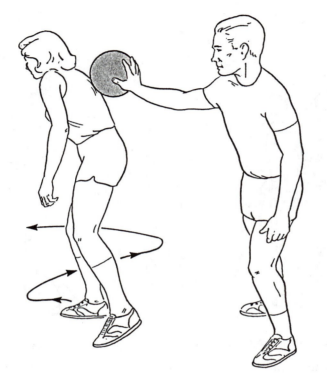

Figure 9-7. Ball on back agility drill with partner.

Purpose: To promote agility and gradually raise the heart rate.

SP: Place the ball on the partner's back with one hand.

ES: The partner with the ball on his back begins *walking*, changing directions frequently, in an attempt to cause the back partner to lose control of the ball that he is holding.

Note: The partner with the ball on his back must *walk slowly*.

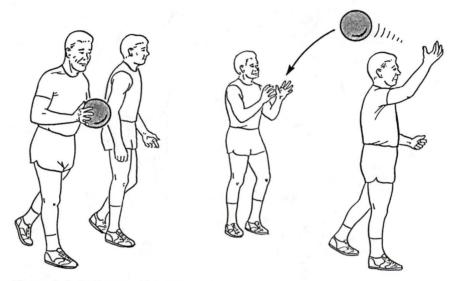

Figure 9–8. Ball toss with partner while walking, alternating positions.

Purpose: To stretch the arm and shoulder muscles and gradually raise the heart rate.

SP: Standing, side-by-side with a partner, with one partner holding a ball as illustrated.

ES: The partner holding the ball walks quickly in front of the other, tossing the ball over his shoulder as shown. The sequence is repeated while both partners continue walking. Alternate use of the left and right arms in the ball toss.

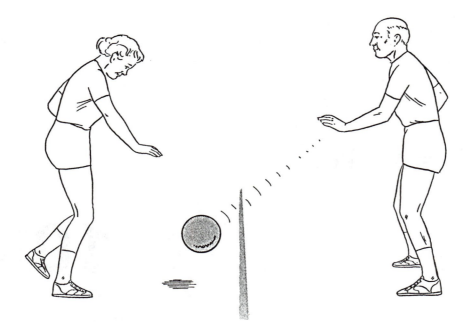

Figure 9–9. Ball volley with partner.

Purpose: To improve hand-eye coordination and gradually raise the heart rate.

SP: Stand about 6 to 8 feet from a partner, using any "line" on the floor to separate the respective courts. One partner holds a volleyball or playground ball.

ES: Volley the ball back-and-forth over the line which is used as an imaginary net. The ball is permitted to bounce once on each court before it is struck with the palm of an open hand. One point is awarded to the server when the ball is not appropriately returned.

Note: The competitive nature of this activity can be modified by encouraging partners to "work together" to see how many consecutive volleys they can accomplish in a given time period (e.g., within one minute). Alternatively, the exercise leader may request that all hits be made with the non-dominant hand, or that the players alternate hands when striking the ball.

10

Group Activities

The following activities, using a playground ball, volleyball, or cage ball, are primarily designed to complement the warm-up, cool-down, and endurance components of the exercise session. For all activities: Purpose = primary reason for activity and/or focus on muscle groups that are employed; SP = starting position; ES = exercise sequence; and, Note = special considerations and/or modifications.

The number of repetitions of each activity or time allotted for them is left to the exercise leader's discretion.

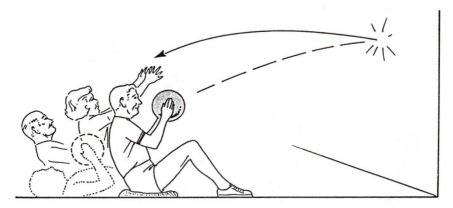

Figure 10-1. Triple sit-up.

Purpose: To develop abdominal muscle tone and timing.

SP: Three or more participants sit side by side facing a wall with legs flexed at the knee joint at a distance of 5 to 6 feet from the wall. One participant is holding a ball.

ES: The participant holding the ball push passes it to the wall. One of the other participants catches the rebounding ball and all three simultaneously do a sit-up movement. Activity continues in the same manner. When timing is perfected, the ball is caught as the participants start to move to the lying position and thrown to the wall as they begin to sit up. If participants are unable to sit up, the movement of chin to chest and shoulders off the floor with arms extended is also effective. For additional variation, the participant tossing the ball can call the name of the designated receiver.

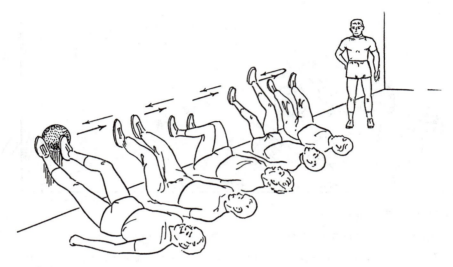

Figure 10–2. Ball on wall agility drill with feet.

Purpose: To improve coordination and tone the muscles of the abdomen.

SP: Approximately 5 to 10 participants lined up shoulder-to-shoulder, lying on the floor, with the knees flexed and feet resting on an adjacent wall.

ES: Pass the ball with the feet from one person to another so that it remains against the wall and travels to the end of the line and back (i.e., to the original starting point). The ball should be maintained between the feet and the wall at all times. If the ball is dropped (i.e., hits the floor) anywhere on route, the exercise leader should place it at the head of the line once again, until the maneuver is successfully completed.

Note: This activity can be easily adapted to a relay format where two teams with an equal number of participants compete to see which one can move the ball down-the-line and back in the fastest time. Once again, if the ball is dropped on route, it is returned to the starting position.

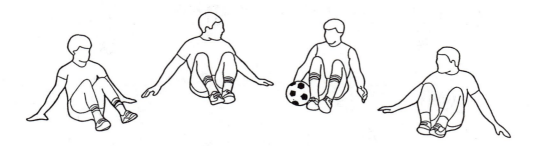

Figure 10–3. Ball roll around circle.

Purpose: To tone and strengthen the abdominal muscles.

SP: This exercise requires several people who are sitting in a circle, facing inward.

ES: The ball is rolled on the floor clockwise or counterclockwise around the circle, under the participants' legs. The feet should be raised off the floor, knees together, as the ball goes under each participant's legs.

Note: Participants should be cautioned to avoid breath-holding during this exercise.

Note: This activity can be modified by having one participant standing outside the circle, directly opposite (i.e., farthest away) from someone seated in the circle who is holding a sport ball. The individuals in the circle try to keep the ball "away from" the person on the outside of the circle by rolling it under the legs, around the circle, in either direction. If the person running around the outside of the circle manages to touch the back of the person with the ball as it is passed under the legs, he/she switches places with the individual in the circle who was touched on the back.

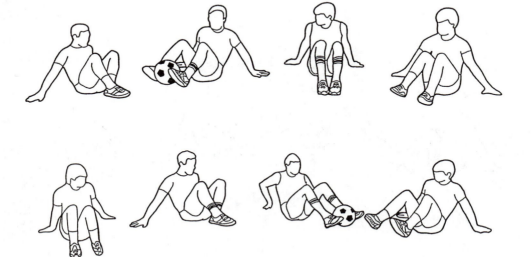

Figure 10–4. Ball passing (with feet) around circle.

Purpose: To tone and strengthen the abdominal muscles.

SP: This exercise requires several people who are sitting in a circle, facing inward.

ES: As the ball is picked up with the feet and held in the air, the participant rotates on his "seat" and places the ball on the floor to the person next to him who continues the sequence.

Note: Participants should be cautioned to avoid breath-holding during this activity. The ball should *not* be passed in mid-air from one participant to another.

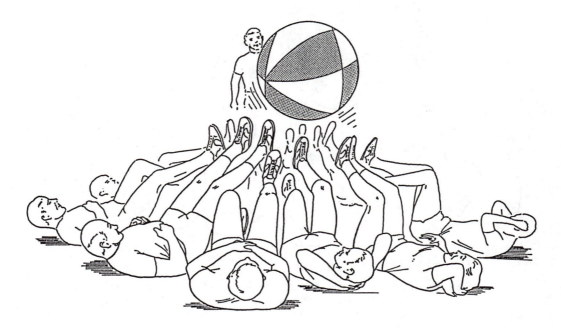

Figure 10–5. Keep the cage ball moving.

Purpose: To stretch and tone the muscles of the legs, lower back, and abdomen. (NOTE: This is an enjoyable and challenging activity that is particularly applicable for the cool-down phase of the execise session. It requires a great deal of teamwork.)

SP: The participants lie on the floor as shown, forming a "tight circle" (i.e., nearly shoulder to shoulder), with the knees flexed, legs raised and lower back in contact with the floor.

ES: The exercise leader places a large cage ball in the center of the circle, on top of the participants feet, and challenges the group to keep the ball moving and in the air with gentle foot tapping, without losing control (i.e., letting the ball fall to the ground outside the circle). Competition can be established by having one group of participants challenge another to see which can keep the ball in the air the longest. Alternatively, the exercise leader may record the time that the ball is maintained in the air, to see if this "record time" can be beaten in future sessions.

Note: The activity can be made even more challenging by requiring the participants to pass one or two small playground balls to the person on their right and/or left while they simultaneously keep the cage ball in motion with their feet.

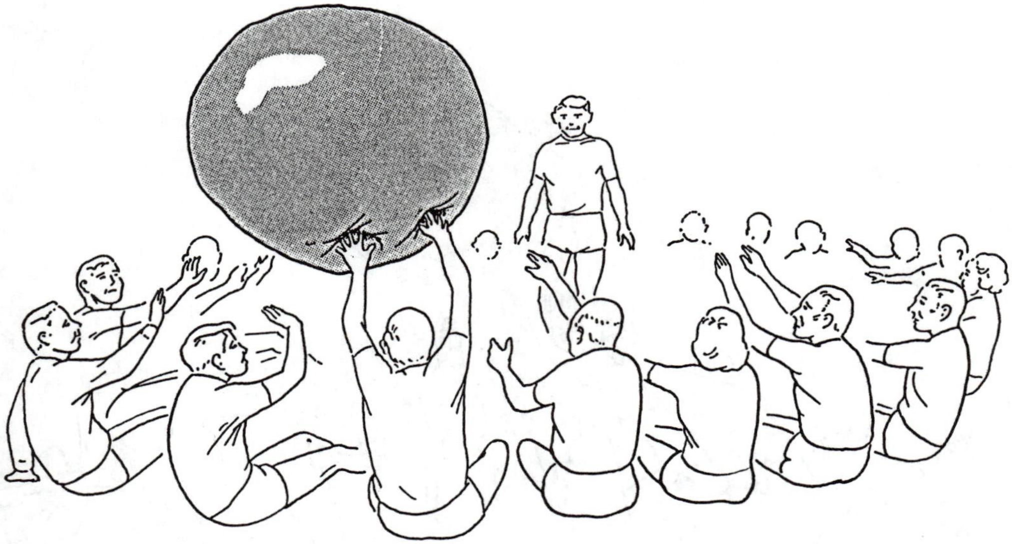

Figure 10-6. Pass the cage ball.

Purpose: To stretch the muscles of the arms and shoulders. (NOTE: This is an enjoyable and challenging activity that is particularly applicable to the cool-down phase of the exercise session. It requires a great deal of teamwork.)

SP: The participants sit on the floor as shown, forming a "tight circle" (i.e., nearly shoulder to shoulder), arms overhead, with the legs outstretched and knees slightly flexed.

ES: The exercise leader places a large cage ball in the center of the circle, resting on the participants' hands, and challenges the group to keep the ball moving and in the air with gentle hand pushing (i.e., either around the circle or back and forth) without allowing the ball to fall to the ground inside or outside the circle. Competition or modifications can be incorporated as described for "keep the cage ball moving."

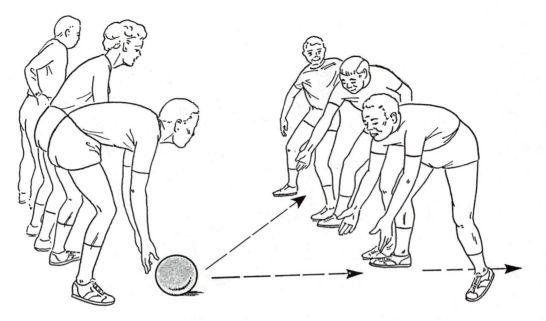

Figure 10–7. Ball roll through opponent's legs.

Purpose: A trunk flexion activity.

SP: Two lines of an equal number of participants face each other at a distance of about 8 to 12 feet. Legs are to be at least shoulder width apart. Sides of participants' feet touch one another.

ES: A ball is rolled with the goal being to successfully get it through the legs of any opponent before it is diverted or stopped with the hands. Feet must remain in place.

Sugges-
tion: Vary distance between participants. Use a varied number and size of sport balls.

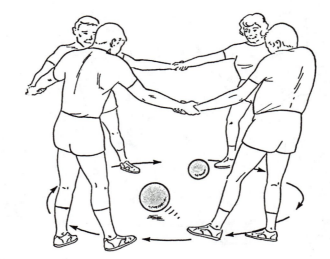

Figure 10-8. Group circling with foot-ball tapping.

Purpose: To promote balance and agility and gradually raise the heart rate.

SP: Using 4 or more participants, form a circle by facing inward and locking wrists. One or 2 playground balls should be placed on the floor in the circle, within footstriking distance.

SE: Initiate a sidestep motion in one direction, while simultaneously tapping the ball(s). The object of the activity is to maintain continuous movement of the participants and playground ball(s), while keeping the ball(s) within the circumference of the circle.

Note: The activity can be modified by having the participants change direction (i.e., sidestepping to the left then sidestepping to the right, or vice versa).

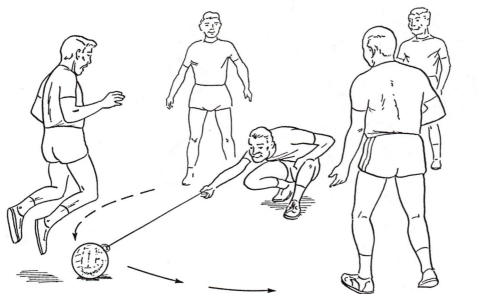

Figure 10-9. Ball jumping.

Purpose: To enhance agility and leg power by timed jumping movements.

SP: A circle of 4 to 10 participants with one person in the circle center.

ES: Person in the center of the circle swings a tethered ball in a 360-degree radius. Each participant jumps over the ball as it approaches them. As skill improves, the height of the arc can be raised to midleg.

Sugges-
tion: A sock filled with rags can be substituted for the tethered ball. To avoid dizziness, the person in the center of the circle can use the right hand for one-half of the arc and switch the rope or line to the opposite hand to complete the 360 degrees.

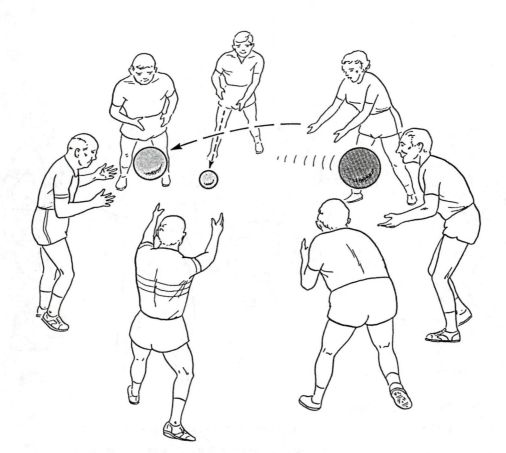

Figure 10-10. Circle pass.

Purpose: To improve hand-eye coordination, gradually increase heart rate, and enhance range of motion.

SP: Several participants form a circle, with 1 or more persons holding a ball.

ES: Pass the ball to anyone in the circle; that person then passes the ball to someone else in the circle; the activity continues by keeping the ball going from person to person.

Note: Encourage the participants to toss the ball in the air and bounce it off the ground.

Note: Increase the number of balls used at one time; use balls of different sizes and weights.

Note: Initially keep the players standing in one spot; then progress by having them circle to the left or right while the ball(s) is (are) being passed.

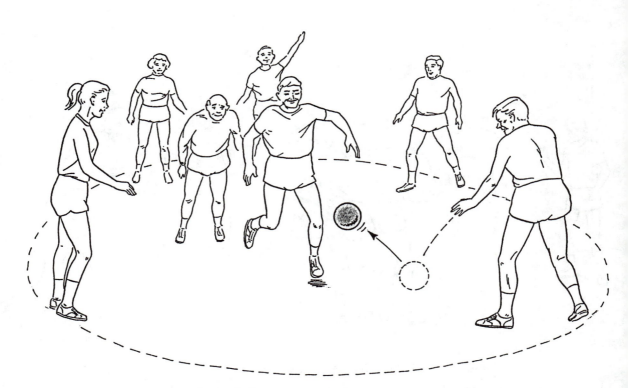

Figure 10-11. Bounce Dodgeball.

Purpose: To practice ball passing skills and agility.

SP: Circle formation with 1, 2, or 3 participants in the circle.

ES: Pass the ball randomly to circle participants with the objective of striking an inner circle member below the waist after a bounce pass. When a hit is made, passer becomes an inner circle member and the participant who was struck joins the outer circle.

Sugges-
tion: Vary type of pass, size of outer circle, number of balls in play.

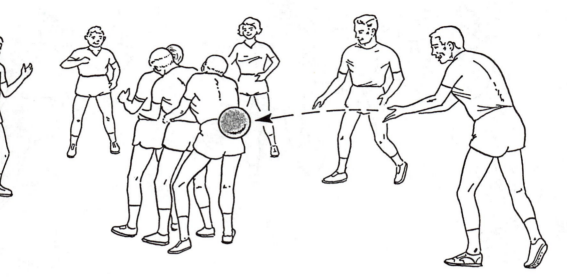

Figure 10-12. Circle — Engine and Caboose.

Purpose: To practice ball passing skills and agility.

SP: Circle formation with 3 participants in the center of the circle. First participant (engine) faces person with the ball, second participant places arms around the waist of first, third participant (caboose) places arms around the waist of the second.

ES: Ball is passed rapidly and randomly about the circle from player to player. The goal is to strike the posterior of the third person (caboose) in the center circle. Moving as a team, the three person unit attempts to avoid the ball contacting the caboose. When a successful hit is made the thrower becomes the caboose and players move up with number one, engine, joining the circle.

Sugges-
tions: Use a variety of passes. Use 2 balls. Size of circle can be varied.

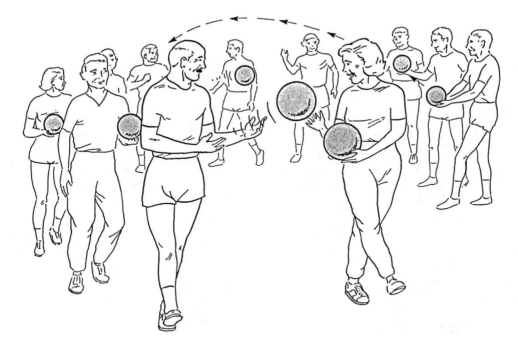

Figure 10-13. Group ball toss or exchange.

Purpose: To improve hand-eye coordination and gradually raise the heart rate.

SP: A group aerobic activity with a large number of participants who are each holding a playground ball.

ES: Participants begin walking in different directions on a large floor. As one individual approaches another he or she should *simultaneously* exchange balls (i.e., either by handing or gently tossing them). The object of this fun activity is to maintain continuous movement of participants and playground balls (i.e., no participant should be holding the same ball for more than 5 seconds).

Note: This activity can be made even more enjoyable by utilizing one ball that is different from all of the others (e.g., a white volleyball amid 15 red playground balls). The exercise leader may, before the activity starts, declare "the winner" to be the person who is holding the volleyball after a designated time (e.g., 60 seconds). The leader keeps track of the time during the activity, yells "stop" when the time is up, and notes "the winner."

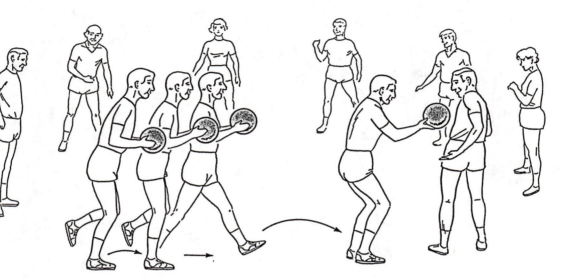

Figure 10-14. Game of spud.

Purpose: A simple low-intensity contest requiring some agility.

SP: Participants circle about one person holding a ball.

ES: The participant holding the ball tosses it vertically upward using a 2-hand underarm motion and calls either a name or number. All participants except the one called walk rapidly away from the tossed ball. When the ball is caught by the "designated" participant, he or she yells, "spud." All participants are to stop and "freeze" in position. The person with the ball must take 1 hop, 1 step, and 1 jump to the closest participant or participant of choice. When possible, the person can be tagged with the ball. If the ball is thrown, it must strike the person below the waist. The person tagged or target of the throw becomes the next person to toss the ball upward and call a name or number. Play continues.

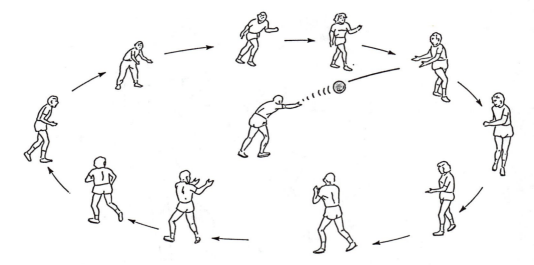

Figure 10-15. Circle ball toss.

Purpose: To improve hand-eye coordination and gradually raise (or lower) heart rate.

SP: Form a large circle with the exercise leader holding a ball while standing in the center of the circle.

ES: The participants begin walking in one direction. They must, however, maintain visual contact with the exercise leader who may throw the ball to them at any time. The participant catches the ball while walking, and throws it back to the exercise leader. The exercise leader can call for a direction change at any time. Competition may be incorporated into the activity by noting how many consecutive tosses can be completed by the group without dropping the ball. Accordingly, records can be established to improve upon at future exercise sessions.

Note: This activity can be made even more challenging by having 2 playground balls moving *simultaneously*. One ball is tossed back-and-forth from the exercise leader to the participants, while the second ball is passed around the circumference of the circle (i.e., over the shoulder to the person behind). If the group is large enough, 2 participants back-to-back, can toss the playground balls to the circle participants. Upon command, ball tossing can be of the following types: behind back, push pass, unpreferred hand only, etc.

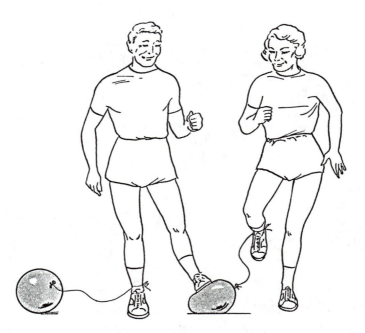

Figure 10-16. Balloon busting contest.

Purpose: To practice abdominal breathing and forced expiration by blowing up a balloon. This game also improves balance and agility.

SP: Standing with an inflated balloon tied to the right ankle at a distance of 24 inches.

ES: Have all participants inflate balloons and tie them to their right ankles. Using a large floor space have participants *walk* as rapidly as possible and attempt to break a fellow participant's balloon. If a person's balloon is busted, he or she is eliminated from the game space. Winner is the last person to have a balloon intact.

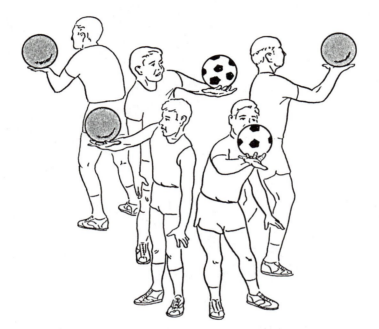

Figure 10-17. Ball balance while walking.

Purpose: To improve balance and coordination and gradually raise the heart rate.

SP: Utilizing a large floor and a number of participants, each individual *balances* a playground ball on the *back* of the hand (fingers and arm outstretched), as shown.

ES: Participants begin walking in different directions while maintaining the ball balanced on the back of the hand. If the opposite hand or chest is used to stabilize the ball, the participant is "out." The last participant remaining is "the winner."

Note: This activity can be made even more challenging (and fun) by encouraging participants to "gently bump" hips as they walk next to each other in an attempt to make someone else drop a ball.

        Another modification of the activity that is even more challenging, is to encourage the participants, when approaching each other, to *simultaneously* toss and exchange balls, while catching them on the back of the hand.

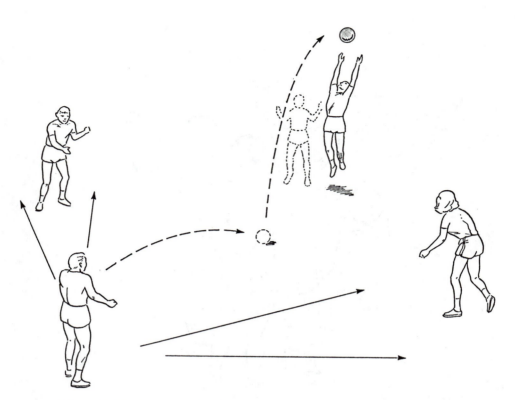

Figure 10-18. Jump and reach.

Purpose: To develop leg power and encourage body extension movements.

SP: Four to 6 participants standing at an equal distance apart (e.g., 12 to 15 feet) from one another.

ES: Person with a ball executes a 2-handed overarm bounce pass to a fellow participant. Bouncing ball height should require the catcher to be air bound with arms at full extension. The catcher bounce passes the ball to another participant.

Sugges-
tion: Use a rubber sport ball to attain the desired bouncing height.

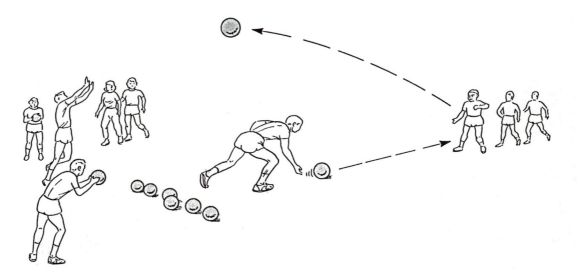

Figure 10-19. Kickball formation drill.

Purpose: To enhance ball kicking and catching skills.

SP: Any area large enough to accommodate 10 to 20 participants. Use 3 participants "at bat," 1 bowler and 5 or more fielders. Bowler should be 20 to 30 feet from kicker. A supply of at least 10 balls can be used.

ES: Bowler rolls ball to kicker. Kicker may kick up to 3 times before becoming a fielder by walking or jogging on to the playing area, to the bowler's extreme left. Fielders constantly move to the bowler's right, assuming new positions as the activity progresses. Farthest participant on the bowler's right joins the kicking group. Caught or retrieved ground balls are relayed to the bowler. Bowler (usually the exercise leader) gets as many balls in play as rapidly as possible. Activity is continuous and kicking legs should be alternated.

11

Recreational Games

The following recreational games, using a playground ball, volleyball, or cage ball, are designed to challenge skill, balance, and agility and complement the endurance phase of the program. For selected games: Purpose = primary reason for activity; SP = starting position; ES = exercise sequence; and, Note = special considerations and/or modifications.

166

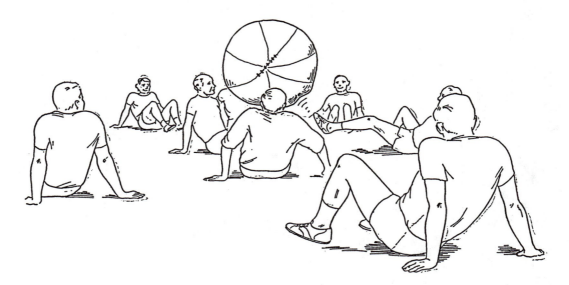

Figure 11-1. Cageball soccer.

Playing
area: A large floor space or basketball court with a rectangular goal at
              each end; goal size 9 to 12 feet in width. Goals may be constructed
              from tape (on a wall), pilons, cages, or floor mats placed against a
              wall.

# of play-
ers: Equal number on each team.

Playing
time: First team to score a designated number of goals, or time arbitrarily
              determined by the exercise leader.

Equip-
ment: Cageball (3 to 5 foot diameter).

Rules/
scoring: All players are in the seated position, hands on the floor for support.
              The game is started by a face-off in the center of the court. The ball
              may be moved with the feet only; hand-ball contact is not permitted.
              The objective is to advance the cageball toward the opponents' goal.
              Contact of the ball with the goal scores a point, followed by a new
              face-off. Player movement up-and-down the court is by crab-walk
              only. Goalies are frequently alternated. There are no out-of-bounds
              since the walls may be used to pass the ball from one player to
              another. The winner is the team with the most goals.

Penalties: A no-hands game. Penalty is charged against team members using
              their hands; the opposing team receives the ball side out.

Note: Participants with arm, wrist or shoulder problems may assist as ref-
              erees.

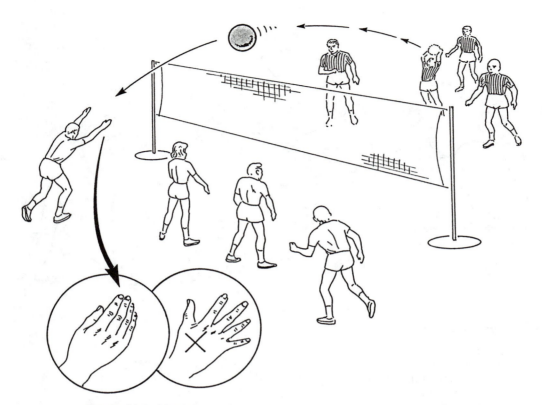

Figure 11-2. Medicine ball over the net.

Purpose: To push and catch a relatively heavy object.

SP: A net of any height, e.g., 5 foot (badminton net), 7 ½, or 8 foot (volleyball net), with at least 2 to 6 participants per side. There are no specific boundary lines. Use a medicine ball weighing approximately 4, 8, or 12 pounds.

ES: Using a variety of pass-type movements, a team member throws the ball over the net by any one of the following: shot put, 2-arms overhead, push pass, or over-the-head using both arms in an underarm throwing movement with back toward net. Receiving team member must catch the medicine ball on the fly or 1 point is scored against them. Game is 5 points. Team position rotates in a counterclockwise direction after each point.

Variations: 1. Medicine ball is passed and caught by each team member before it is tossed over the net.

2. The medicine ball receiver must execute a 360-degree turn before passing the ball to a team member or over the net.

Note: The medicine ball is caught with the thumb along the medial aspect of the palm of the hand and touching the index finger (see illustration). Fingers are flexed. Ball contact is made at the abdomen by having the arms rapidly adducting.

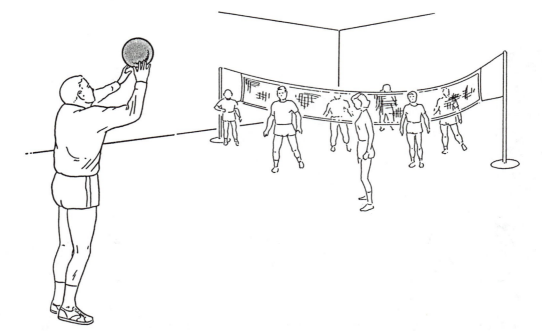

Figure 11-3. One-bounce volleyball.

Playing
area: Volleyball court with a net height between 6 and 8 feet.

\# of Play-
ers: Any number may play; generally 5 to 9 players per side. When a team
has a player talent advantage, the exercise leader should move selected players to the opposing side to equalize playing ability between the teams.

Equip-
ment: Volleyball

Rules/
scoring: The game is started by a volley-for-serve during which the ball must
cross the net a minimum of 3 times. The winner of the volley gains
the right to serve first. Standard volleyball rules are followed *except*
one or more floor bounces and as many as 3 hits per side are permitted, as established by the exercise leader. (Allowing one or more
bounces of the ball per side facilitates longer play and provides additional fun, while minimizing the skill level required to play the game.)
Failure to return the ball over the net results in a loss of service. A
point is scored when the serving team returns the ball over the net
one more time than the opponent. Player rotation can occur after
each point or service.

Penalties: Side out is declared when the ball is struck more than 1 time in succession by a single player, or more than 3 times in succession by a
team.

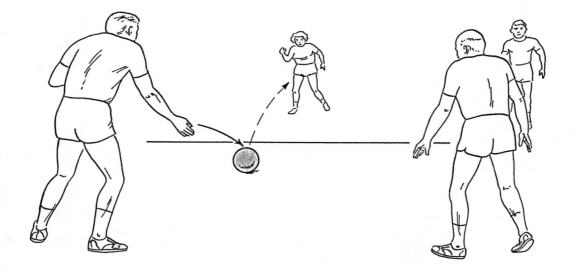

Figure 11-4. Bounceball.

This activity has some aspects of tennis and volleyball. It can be played with a minimum of 2 players, a bounce ball, and a flat surface. There are no set boundaries; the particular area defines the boundaries or they can be pre-determined, e.g., a volleyball court.

Purpose: To keep the ball in play for as long as possible to ensure a controlled elevation in heart rate.

SP/ES: 1) The basic format of bounce ball is that the ball is hit by one player to another player with a bounce between players.

2) A center line separates the area into 2 courts or sides. A center line could be adhesive tape, an extended rope placed on the floor, or a bench or some other low barrier above ground. The ball must bounce on the hitter's side of the court and can bounce once between players on the other side before being returned. The ball must be bounced in the hitter's court before it passes over the center line or barrier to the opponent's side.

3) Players can be added to each side.

4) Limits to the number of players who must touch the ball before it is bounced over the center line or barrier can be established. The more players, the slower the game (participation); the fewer players, the faster the game (competition).

5) As skill progresses, the ball does not have to bounce when passed between players on one side but must still be hit to bounce off the ground immediately before going over the center line to the other side.

Scoring: A point is scored when: A) the ball does not strike the hitter's court before bouncing over the center line or barrier, B) the ball cannot be successfully returned by an opposing team or opponent, C) more than 1 bounce occurs before the ball is passed or struck.

Only the serving side can score a point. Game is 5 to 10 points. Participants rotate in a clockwise or counterclockwise direction upon a change in serve, similar to volleyball.

Note: Bounceball can accommodate many players. It can have many variations and is adaptable to all skill levels.

1) It can be played with as few as 2 players and an almost unlimited number if the playing surface is large enough.

2) The participation by players is controllable. For a large group, insist that at least 3 players touch the ball on each side before it is bounced back to the other side.

3) The skill level of players can be accommodated by insisting the ball bounce between players on one side or by keeping the ball off the ground when it is passed and insisting that the only time the ball bounces is as it is returned to the other side.

4) Variations include using the unpreferred hand in passing or striking the ball.

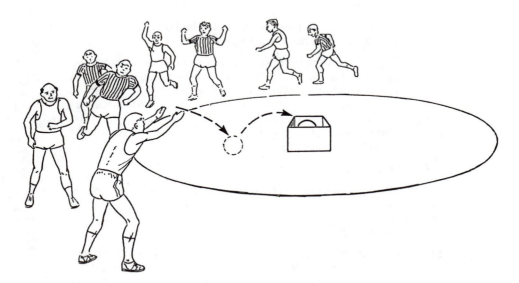

Figure 11-5. Boxball.

Playing
area: A team game with a large open box as a goal which is secured in the middle of a circle drawn on the floor some distance from the box. Participants cannot step into the circle.

\# of Play-
ers: Any number may play; generally 3 to 6 players per side.

Equip-
ment: Sportball or volleyball.

Rules/
scoring: The object of the game is for the team to bounce the ball into the box (which scores 1 point) as many times as possible in a given time period. The basic format is where the defenders try to stop the offensive players from scoring (e.g., by intercepting the ball). To control the intensity of the activity, the number of players can be increased or decreased. The number of players who must bounce the ball or to whom the ball can be passed before a goal can be attempted can be increased or decreased. To accommodate different skill levels, specific regulations can be incorporated. for example, a) the ball must bounce when passed, or b) the ball must be caught and thrown with only one hand.

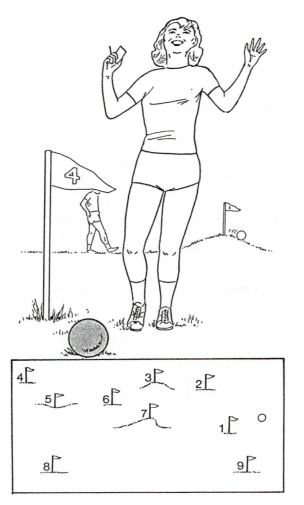

Figure 11-6. Kick ball golf.

Playing
area: Any grassy outdoor area (80 to 300 yards). The size of the area is not
            important. The ideal playing area might include a water hazard,
            small rolling hills as well as level terrain, trees, telephone poles, or
            implanted utility poles.

# of play-
ers: Any number of players can be involved. There may be individual,
            partner, or team play.

Playing
time: Determined by the exercise leader.

Equip-
ment: A wide variety of sport balls (e.g., volleyball, soccer ball) may be
            used. An inflated rubber playground ball (8 to 12 inches in diameter)
            is ideal.

(*continued on page 174*)

Figure 11-6. (continued)

Rules/
scoring: Rules are similar to conventional golf, except that sport balls and wooden stakes (holes) are employed. Cardboard or cloth flags designating the hole number may be mounted at the top of each wooden stake. The number of holes is determined by the exercise leader, as is the arbitrarily established tee for each hole. The success of the game depends on the exercise leader's ability to create a golf course that is interesting and challenging. Many variations are possible: dog legs, water hazards, or placing the stakes on hilly terrain. Before the players tee off, the leader determines the par for the hole by evaluating the distance and hazards that may be encountered. Example: a 200-yard hole might be considered a par 5, while a 60-yard hole may be a par 3. The ball may be kicked from the ground, dropkicked, or punted; *players must walk briskly or jog between kicks*. The object of the game is to strike the wooden stake (hole) in the fewer number of strokes. Individual scores may be recorded on real golf cards. The tee for the next hole is adjacent to the hole that was just completed. The lowest score on a predetermined number of holes constitutes the winner.

Varia-
tions: When teams of 4 members or more are possible, the team plays the best ball. If there are insufficient numbers of sportballs available, team members alternate turns kicking and walking briskly together. Unpreferred kicking legs can be used or the last shot to the hole could be bowled using the left or right arm.

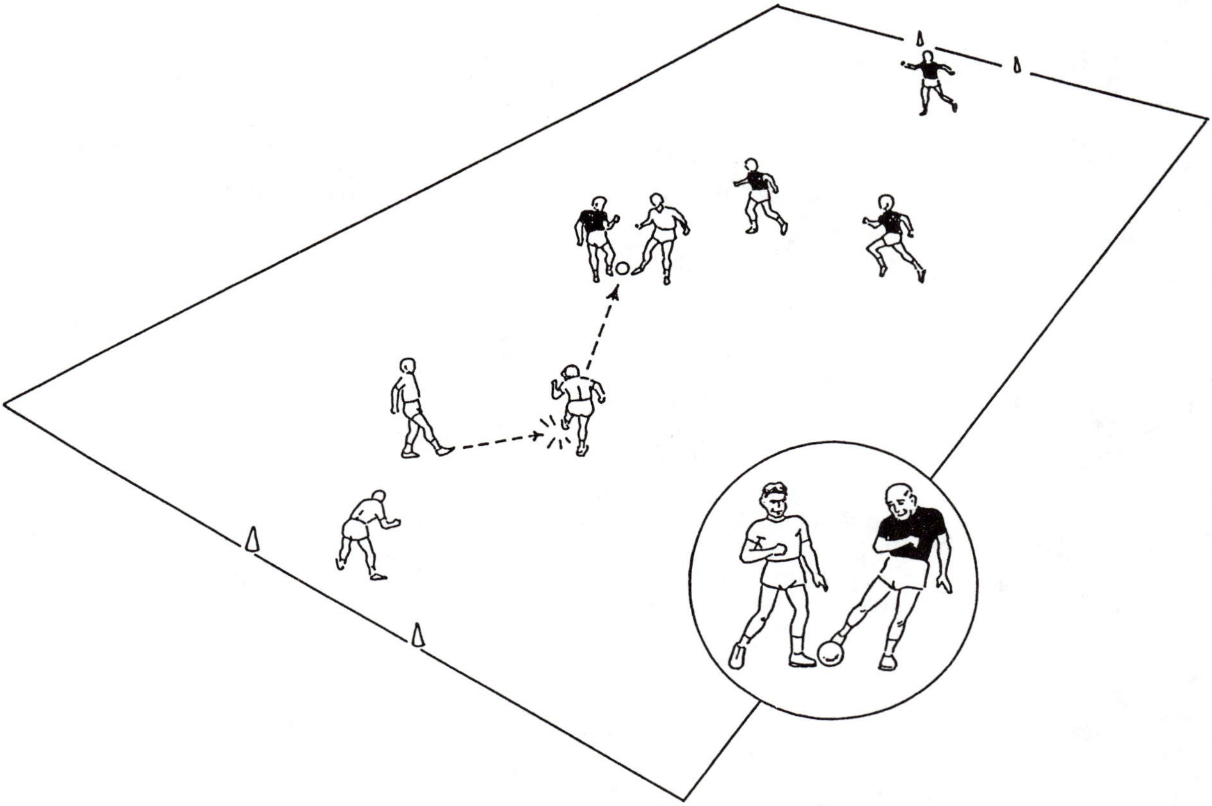

Figure 11-7. Walking-soccer activity.

Purpose: A moderate intensity intermittent activity to stimulate the heart and circulatory system and to practice agility skills.

SP: An indoor or outdoor playing surface with boundary lines and two 10-foot wide goals identified by road cones. There should be an equal number of players on each side with a goalie for each team.

ES: Ball is advanced by a foot dribble and passed to team members as defensive players impede progress toward goal. A goal is scored when the ball is kicked past the goalie through the goal area (i.e., road cones). No physical contact is permitted.

Defensive team members should remain at least 1 yard (3 feet) from their opponents. Out-of-bounds or participant contact fouls are called by team members. Change goalies frequently and sustain play for 5 to 10 minutes.

Note: Participant heart rate checks should be done periodically during the game. To prevent the exercise intensity from becoming too high, jogging or running should be prohibited and appropriately penalized (e.g., free kick for opposing team).

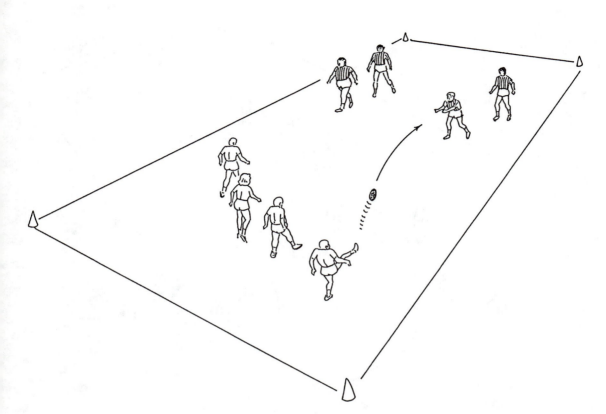

Figure 11-8. Touch football-passing only game.

Purpose: To stimulate the heart and circulatory system and encourage team play.

SP: Any indoor or outdoor playing space with boundary lines identified by road cones. There should be an equal number of team members on each side.

ES: Ball (volleyball, football, sport ball) is kicked to a receiving team. *Walking only* is permitted to advance or defend. Passing the ball is permitted forward, backward, or laterally at any time. When the person with the ball is touched, the play stops. After a huddle, a team is allowed a maximum of 3 downs in which to score a touchdown. If the team is unsuccessful in scoring, the ball is taken over by the opposing team.

Play continues for 5 to 10 minutes with heart rates checked at least once.

Note: This activity is essentially traditional "touch football" with 3 major modifications: first, only walking is permitted; second, only passing is allowed (either forward, backward or laterally); and third, only 3 downs are allowed in which to score a touchdown.

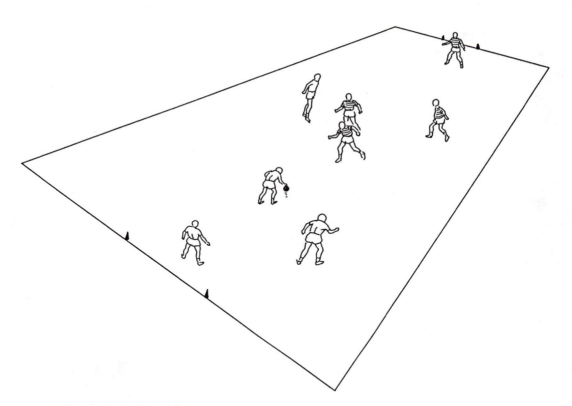

Figure 11-9. 3×3×3 Game.

Purpose: An aerobic game to practice motor coordination skills.

SP: An identifiable field of play, gymnasium space, or outdoors, with
        boundaries marked with road cones. A goal 10 feet in width is placed
        on the end line using road cones. An equal number of players are on
        each side with one player of each team serving as goalie.

ES: A ball is moved forward toward an opponent's goal. Fast walking is
        recommended. The advancing team member is allowed to hold the
        ball for 3 seconds, take 3 steps, or execute 3 ground dribbles. Any or
        all of the 3×3×3 can be performed before the ball is passed to a team
        member. All defensive efforts must include walking only and *no*
        physical contact. A goal is scored when a player *bowls* the ball past
        the goalie through the goal area. The team having been scored
        against advances the ball toward the opponent's goal. Rules are kept
        to a minimum. For out-of-bounds infractions, the team last touching
        the ball becomes the defensive team as ball possession changes. An
        additional safety rule is to keep defensive players at least 1 yard (3
        feet) from the opponent. As a variation to scoring, the ball may be
        kicked on the ground past the goalie through the goal area. An ade-
        quate playing time is from 5 to 10 minutes. Check heart rates at least
        1 time during play.

12

Relays

The following relays, using a playground ball or volleyball, are designed to challenge skill, balance, and agility and complement the endurance phase of the program. For all relays: Purpose = primary reason for activity; SP = starting position; ES = exercise sequence; and, Note = special considerations and/or modifications.

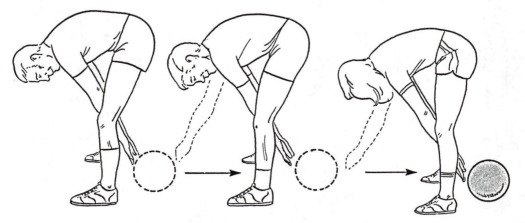

Figure 12-1. Ball between leg relay.

Purpose: Increase range of motion and increase heart rate.

SP: Participants stand in a file; number of participants determines the intensity of the relay.

ES: The ball is passed from first in file to last in file between each participant's legs. The last person brings ball to the front of the file. Process is repeated so that everyone gets an opportunity to carry the ball to the front of the file.

Note: Alternatively, the ball can be moved from the last to the first person. Ball may be bounced, soccer dribbled, soccer headed, or kicked while moving to starting position.

Note: The exercise leader can turn this relay into a contest between 2 or more teams with equal numbers of participants.

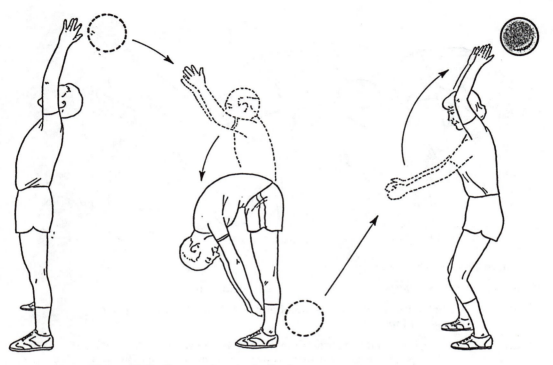

Figure 12-2. Over and under ball relay.

Purpose: Increase range of motion and increase heart rate.

SP: Participants stand in a file; number of participants determines the
        intensity of the relay. The first participant in the file (i.e., at the head
        of the line) is holding a ball overhead.

ES: Pass ball to back of file over head/under legs. See "Ball between leg
        relay" for possible ways to continue the relay.

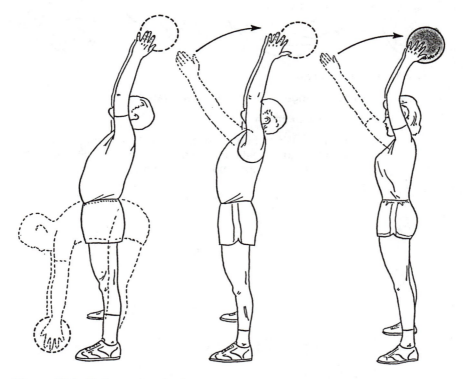

Figure 12-3. Ball over head relay.

Purpose: Increase range of motion and increase heart rate.

SP: As in figure and as described in "Ball between leg relay."

ES: Pass ball from front to back of file over head. See description in "Ball
           between leg relay" for possible ways to modify the relay.

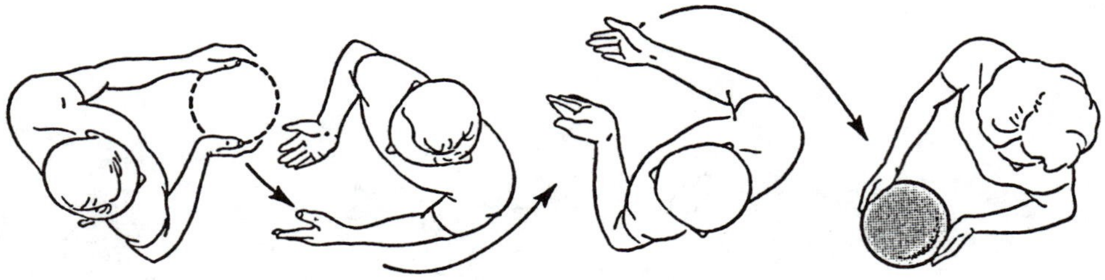

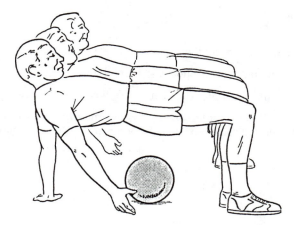

Figure 12-4. Figure-8 relay.

Purpose: To increase range of motion and heart rate.

SP: Stand in file with ball in front.

ES: Rotating the trunk alternately to right and left, handing off the ball to the person behind so that it moves to the back of the file. See "Ball between leg relay" for possible ways to continue the relay.

Figure 12-5. Bridge ball relay.

Purpose: To tone muscles of the abdomen and increase heart rate.

SP: Start as in "Bridge Ball" but in file next to each other.

ES: Pass ball from front to back of file as shown. When ball is through bridge, sit until ball comes back. See "Ball between leg relay" for possible ways to continue the relay.

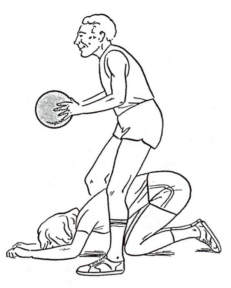

Figure 12-6. Over back relay.

Purpose: To enhance agility and increase the heart rate.

SP: Participants kneel in a file, facing the floor, with the back rounded and forearms on the ground. The last person in line is standing, holding a ball, with the feet slightly more than shoulder width apart.

ES: The person standing carries the ball to the front of the file by straddling the other participants, as shown. Before this person assumes a kneeling position, like the others, he throws or rolls the ball to the individual who is now standing at the end of the file. The relay continues until everyone has had the opportunity to move from last to first in the file.

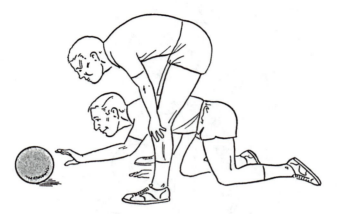

Figure 12-7. Ball push between leg relay.

Purpose: To enhance agility and increase the heart rate.

SP: Participants stand in a file, leaning forward, with the feet spread apart and hands on the knees. The last person in line is on "all fours," holding a ball.

ES: The crawler pushes the ball between the participants' legs to the front of the file. As this person assumes a standing position, he throws or rolls the ball to the individual who is now at the end of the file. The relay continues until everyone has had an opportunity to move from last to first in the file.

13

Summary

Despite the increasing body of scientific evidence documenting the benefits of regular aerobic exercise, greater public interest in fitness than ever before, and the claim that exercise may have "addictive properties,"[3] only 1 in 5 Americans gets regular, vigorous exercise.[4] While many individuals can be motivated to take the first step toward an exercise commitment, few sustain the interest and enthusiasm needed to maintain participation.

Exercise must be recognized as a lifetime pursuit and not merely a "program" of 10 or 12 weeks duration that will have lasting benefits. To this end, the individual must develop an attitude toward exercise that reinforces adherence. Probably the single most important factor shaping this attitude is the well-trained exercise leader.[5] But perhaps equally important are the leader's intangible characteristics — contagious enthusiasm, imagination, and excellent people-management skills, all of which are vital to sustain interest and maintain long-term participation.

Exercise leaders should develop programs that are safe, effective, and enjoyable. Leaders should educate and motivate participants.[1] The principles, ideas, and activities described in this book can help to achieve these objectives. We have used them over the years with good adherence in our adult fitness[6] and cardiac rehabilitation programs. Nevertheless, these program suggestions and aerobic activities, or modifications of them, can also be used with children, senior adults, or the wheelchair-confined, and in the exercise programming of a broad spectrum of patients, including those with peripheral vascular disease, obesity, diabetes, and chronic obstructive pulmonary disease.[2]

The beauty of the "Games-as-Aerobics" approach is that it maximizes group support and camaraderie by using sports equipment (e.g., balls) in creative activities or game situations that emphasize cooperation (rather than competition), fun, variety, and success. We acknowledge, however, that all of the exercises described in this book are not appropriate for all persons. Thus, exercise leaders should select or modify those activities best suited to the cardiovascular and musculoskeletal conditions of the participants.

In closing, we sincerely hope that the aerobic activities described in this book will not merely be adopted or copied by exercise leaders, but that they will be amplified, modified, and improved — yielding literally thousands of variations to the themes that have been presented.

The challenge is yours! Have fun!

P.S. — If you have developed and field tested an innovative activity that we have omitted, contact us. It will appear in the 2nd edition.

The Authors.

BIBLIOGRAPHY

1. Franklin, B. (1978) "Motivating and Educating Adults to Exercise." *J. Phys. Ed. Rec.* 49:13-17.
2. Franklin, B., S. Gordon, and G.C. Timmis (eds.). (1989) *Exercise in Modern Medicine*. Williams and Wilkins: Baltimore.
3. Glasser, W. (1976) Positive Addiction. Harper and Row.
4. Lippert, J. (1987) "You Can Make Exercise Fun." *Readers Digest*, August, 108-112.
5. Oldridge, N. (1977) "What to Look For in an Exercise Class Leader." *Phys. Sportsmed.*, 5:85-88.
6. Stoedefalke, K.G. (1974) "Physical Fitness Program for Adults." *Am. J. Cardiol.*, 33:787-790.

ACTIVITIES INDEX

187